Mary Tocco's

MW01537039

Natural Immune Development

A Deeper Understanding of Our Immune System

Mary Tocco

Mary Tocco's Wholistic Heritage Series

Natural Immune Development
A Deeper Understanding of Our Immune System

Editing assistance by Lia Tocco-Miller, DC

Cover design by Austin A. Tocco

Published by Precious Health Campaign LLC

www.ChildhoodShots.com

This book is intended for educational purposes only with the purpose of supplying critical information on the benefits of natural immunity. This information is not to be construed as medical advice. I am not a doctor, nor do I give medical advice. It is up to the individual to make informed healthcare decisions.

This book is dedicated to the memory of my mother,
Viola Marie (Wells) Kosloskey
September 6th, 1924 – April 2nd, 2018

My mother was a true inspiration to me and many others. She was gifted with the ability to see beauty in all of nature and expressed her love for God in her daily life. She taught me compassion for those less fortunate, to accept those different than me, gratitude for my many blessings and most importantly, love for all of God's creations.

Born in Detroit, MI, my mother was raised during the Great Depression. She experienced hunger, poverty and suffered the loss of her mother to cancer when she was 16 years old; leaving her to care for her four younger siblings. Despite early hardships, she mothered eleven children, of which I am number seven.

Her nickname was "Dina", short for Dynamite. Not only was she a strong and independent thinker, but also a beautiful and magnetic woman who turned every head when she entered a room. She encouraged her children to challenge the status quo, ask the hard questions, and stand up for what we believe in—even if our beliefs were considered politically incorrect. No matter what challenges she faced, she always had a positive attitude and looked for the good in people. Long before it was popular or mainstream, Dina embraced natural healthcare and alternative practices. I have her to thank for leading me to chiropractic and holistic health. At her knees I learned to pray, to live by faith, and to trust God in all things.

She was my best friend.

Table of Contents:

"Take no part in the unfruitful works of darkness, but instead expose them." -Ephesians 5:11

Chapter 1

The Vitalistic Philosophy

A question I frequently pose at lectures and in conversations is, "Are we born flawed"? "Did God forget to equip the human body with a fully functioning immune system capable of fighting and overcoming illness"? "Is man fully capable of determining what is needed for human survival"? Every year, things that were considered true in the medical and scientific community prove to be false. Our understanding of the human body is minimal. Humans and animals have lived on Earth for thousands of years, so what role has medical intervention really played? Although, I don't have all the answers, I believe asking these hard questions is important.

I believe God created the human body complete with an immune system designed to protect us throughout life. My beliefs are based on what I call a 'vitalistic' philosophy. This belief is founded on the understanding that the human body has a built-in intelligence called *innate wisdom* which can perform miraculous tasks such as taking two cells (sperm and egg) and create a human being. Even atheists and agnostics can see the visible results of this powerful life-force that gives life order and energy. It is this same intelligence that knows when a wound needs healing, tells the heart to beat, and allows life to thrive in perfect balance with millions of intricacies. In the same manner that an infant is designed with two eyes, a nose, and ten fingers and toes, the infant is also designed with an immune system that is intended to serve and sustain that child for a lifetime.

There is no short cut to natural immune development—a process that begins only five weeks after conception. The natural immune development process involves three major steps. First, natural (wild) exposure to germs and illnesses, second, the subsequent symptoms (body signals) and final stage is natural recovery, all designed to develop the immune system the way humans did for centuries and the way animals adapt in the wild. We must assume that the newborn infant is equipped to do this from birth forward unless there is an obvious congenital abnormality. Even then, the immune system is designed to develop in combat and to avoid this process has consequences.

Step two of the natural immune development process (symptoms) can sometimes be painful, inconvenient, and ever scary. If one does not understand the specifics of what the body is working through, many times trusting the body's innate wisdom and tapping into the vitalistic philosophy can help move through the challenges of symptoms. The vitalist tries not to interfere with the body's innate wisdom and encourages the body to function the way in which it was created. This does not mean that a vitalist is anti-medical nor are they against the use of medications. The vitalist acknowledges the importance of medical intervention in cases of crisis care and emergencies. For example, when my athletic son broke his arm twice while skateboarding, it was obvious we needed to seek emergency care. I felt quite grateful for the skilled orthopedic doctor who set the bones. This is a real-life example of the importance and need for medical intervention

This differs greatly with the practice of medicating children for every symptom and vaccinating for supposed disease prevention. I am of firm belief that medications should be considered a last resort, even when dealing with the symptoms of acute illnesses such as: The flu, colds, swollen glands, measles, chickenpox, whooping cough, mumps and other childhood illnesses.

This vitalistic approach is often difficult to grasp for people who were raised in the traditional medical model of care. The traditional medical model commonly provides a drug for every symptom, and by doing so, many times interferes with the body's natural process of immune development. Medical professionals practice allopathy—eliminating the symptoms of an ailment through chemical intervention, i.e. drugs. One of the problems with allopathy is that it does not address the underlying cause of symptoms—symptoms which are often part of the body's natural defenses. For example, if a child has a headache, the child is given pain medication to reduce the pain with little regard as to the cause of the headache. If a child has a fever, medication is prescribed to reduce the fever with no regard to what is causing the fever and the function of a fever. Allopathy at its core does not treat the body as an intricately connected organism. Each part of the body is viewed as a separate entity, with the focus being the reduction of symptoms. It is common practice to simply mask symptoms with medications and surgeries.

It is not my intention to offend or disrespect those in the medical profession. In many cases, medication possesses the ability to save and extend lives. Modern medicine is quite impressive in many ways. No one can deny the skill required and necessity of a trauma surgeon working on someone who has been seriously injured. Or the essential need of the medical community when someone needs an organ transplant, heart surgery, or medication to control seizures and diabetes, to name a few. Medical practices are truly amazing at helping those in crisis; however, they fail miserably at maintaining health and addressing chronic illnesses.

In most, if not all ways, the vitalistic philosophy is in complete opposition to the traditional medical approach for disease prevention. I believe drug intervention should be a last resort after all other options have been exhausted.

The immune system, like all other systems of the body, is not fully developed at birth. According to modern immunologists, it takes approximately seven to ten years for the immune system to become fully efficient. Medications given frequently to treat normal childhood ailments may result in an immune system that is not yet fully equipped to protect when challenged by serious illnesses.

The vitalistic approach is not for those seeking a short-cut through natural immune development. This approach is often not the easiest nor the most convenient but allowing the immune system to be challenged and develop without intervention pays life-long dividends. This process of natural immune development rewards those who understand and value the way God meant for us to live and thrive. I find that the more one understands natural immunity and how the body works to heal and protect, the less one will fear illness and depend on medications. Just like any parent, it took me a while to trust the body and the healing cycle that must happen when a child is going through what I call "immune system aerobics."

As I present the following Immune System Concepts, I will be referencing concepts developed by immunologist and chiropractor, Dr. Stephen Marini.

In 1976, Dr. Marini received a master's degree in microbiology and Immunology from Hahnemann Medical College in Philadelphia. He then received a Ph.D in Microbiology from the Wistar Institute in Philadelphia. And in 1988, his Doctor of Chiropractic degree from Pennsylvania College of Chiropractic in 1988. Currently, he practices with his son, Dr. Nicholas, in King of Prussia and Philadelphia. Dr. Marini is on the Boards of the International Chiropractic Pediatric Association (ICPA), the Holistic Pediatric Association (HPA) and the Integrated Healthcare Policy Consortium (IHPC). Dr. Marini has a unique understanding of the immune system he calls 'psychoneuroimmunology'.

I've had the pleasure of attending numerous lectures conducted by Dr. Marini's and he's graciously allowed me to pick his brain on several occasions. I first met him over 20 years ago at a chiropractic conference where he presented a lecture on the fundamental components of the immune system. I once again attended a lecture of his in 2007 at a conference I co-hosted called: Hope for Autism and The International Vaccine Symposium. I've also interviewed him on my radio show, 'Healing Our World' on the Republic Broadcasting Network in 2013 and in 2014. He is an exceptional doctor who has been trained in conventional medicine but believes and practices as a vitalist. I've integrated much of his information into my lectures so that people can fully understand the concepts of natural immunity. Throughout this book I will be quoting him from my interviews (in italics) and then elaborating with additional information.

Throughout this book I will also feature the work of immunologist, Tetyana Obukhanych, PhD. She left the world of university research to enlighten people on ways to support a healthy immune system. As someone who was in vaccine research and development for many years, her insights are extremely helpful. Dr. Tetyana says of the modern paradoxical approach to the study of immunology: "Immunology does not study immunity. Immunology studies how the immune system responds to immunization…" She now focuses on nutrition, chiropractic and natural ways to support the immune system so that it can effectively fight and protect as designed.

Chapter 2

The Evolving Scientific View of the Immune System

The study of vaccines or 'Vaccinology' is based on outdated information from the early 1900s. Historically, Immunologists were taught the immune system was a separate part of the body and is isolated. They believed the immune system was autonomous or self-governing and independent of any other part of the body.

They thought the only thing that would respond to the virus in the vaccine was this "isolated" immune system with no regard for how the viruses or other ingredients would affect the immune system, nervous system, brain, organs and tissue in the rest of the body. This would be like saying that when we eat, the only thing that will be affected is the stomach!

This idea lasted until the 1980s when aggressive research into AIDS resulted in the discovery that the immune system is intricately connected to the nervous system. Reported in the Lancet Medical Journal, "The focus of science has shifted from separate entities of the immune system to an interactive immune model.

The foundation of vaccinology (stimulating the immune system chemically to induce a response) is based on archaic information. It is now understood that many organs and bodily systems are involved in immune function: The gut associated lymphoid tissue referred to as GALT, the lympho-epithelial structures of the upper respiratory tract, such as tonsils, and bronchus-associated lymphoid tissue referred to as

BALT. An important basis for local immunity is the migration of specific B and T cells from GALT and BALT to various secretory tissues such as the gut mucosa, the innermost layer of the intestinal tract.

In an article featured in Scientific American, titled "Meet Your Interstitium, A Newfound 'Organ,'" Dr. Neil Theise, professor at NYU's Langone School of Medicine, describes the fluid filled spaces that were found in the body's connective tissues. As written in the article:

Previously, researchers had thought these tissue layers were a dense "wall" of collagen—a strong structural protein found in connective tissue. But the new finding reveals that, rather than a "wall," this tissue is more like an "open, fluid-filled highway." [1]

This "open, fluid-filled highway" involves the connective tissue all over the body, including below the skin; lining the lungs and digestive tract, the urinary system and the surrounding muscles. This new discovery demonstrates the vast complexities of the human body further proving our minimal understanding of the body. This medical discovery should be eye opening and humbling to every doctor. It seems almost unbelievable that in this day in age we are still uncovering enormous findings related to the human body. Our knowledge of the human body is improving every day, but we're nowhere remotely near complete understanding of it.

The immune system is intricately connected to the entire body. For instance, the immune system works with both the

---

[1] Rettner, Rachel. "Meet Your Interstitium, a Newfound 'Organ.'" *Scientific American.* March 27, 2018.

lymphatic and circulatory system to help transport pathogens to immune organs so that the immune system can eradicate them. It also works with the appendix and tonsils which belong to the digestive system. These components of the digestive system help differentiate between pathogens and food which is extremely important for the normal functioning of the immune system. The immune system even works with the skeletal system as it uses blood cells produced by the skeletal system as a method of transportation. The respiratory system, endocrine system and the integumentary system are also involved with immune function. Even the best immunologists admit that we do not have total understanding of all the mechanisms of action…but I assure you, innate intelligence does.

There was a time in history when the words bacteria and virus did not exist. This was pre-1920s before high-powered microscopes were created and modern utilities such as chlorinated running water in the home, toilets, septic fields and sewer systems, soap and antiseptics, and refrigeration were in use. All of which prevent the growth of disease-causing microorganisms.

From the late 1800's to the early 1920's, the death rate was high due to various infectious illnesses. According to the World Health Statistics Annual, 1973-1976: "There has been a steady decline of infectious diseases in most developing countries regardless of the percentage of vaccines administered. The decline was linked to improved sanitation, improved public water supplies, improved personal hygiene and better distribution and increased consumption of fresh fruits and vegetables. In addition, diseases for which there was never a vaccine also declined dramatically."[2] Many diseases, like Scurvy, dysentery and other intestinal infections have significantly reduced due to improved sanitation and nutrition—with no help from a vaccination. In 1948, Congress signed the Federal Water Pollution Control Act providing comprehensive planning, technical services, research, and financial assistance from the federal government to state and local governments for sanitary infrastructure. Other diseases such as Scarlet fever and Tuberculosis have also disappeared without the use of a vaccine.

The first large polio vaccine program was launched by President Theodore Roosevelt in 1954. This program took many years to fully implement, but by the early 1960's school-age children across the U.S. were given polio vaccines via shots or the polio sugar cube. I can vividly remember this time, being in kindergarten and receiving the polio sugar cube. What is rarely discussed is the fact that the death rate from polio had already declined decades before the first vaccine was introduced. The study, "Medical Measures to the Decline of Mortality in the United States in the Twentieth Century" was conducted in 1977 and had the astonishing conclusion that, "Only 3.5% of decline in mortality could be attributed to medical measures." Much of the decline in mortality was in response to improved sanitation and clean water, not medical measures such as vaccinations. This study not only looked at polio but also ten other infectious illnesses.

Modern Immunologist, Tetyana Obukhanych worked at prominent immunology laboratories affiliated with Harvard Medical School and Stanford University School of Medicine.

---

[2] World Health Statistics Annual, 1973-1976, Volume 2. "Diseases on the Way out, Epidemics Have their own Lifespan." 1976.

While on maternity leave, she decided to look deeper into the topic of vaccines. In her E-Book, "Vaccine Illusion", she concludes: "After years of doing research in immunology, observing scientific activities of my superiors, and analyzing vaccine issues, I realized that vaccination is one of the most deceptive inventions that science could ever convince the world to accept. It is not immunity that we gain via vaccination but a puny surrogate of immunity. For this reason, vaccination at its core is neither a safe nor an effective method of disease prevention."[3]

Science is ever evolving, and new concepts, theories and discoveries occur every day. What is considered an absolute truth in science one day may be considered outdated and incorrect the next. It was commonly believed until the 1980's that the brains of infants weren't developed enough to process pain. Because of this false conclusion, most medical procedures performed on infants prior to this time were performed free of anesthesia. Other medical procedures that we once commonly used as a standard of care include lobotomies to treat mental illnesses, the use of tapeworms for weight loss, and bloodletting to prevent and treat diseases (which is what killed President George Washington). I would estimate that medical professionals might feel mortified when looking back at some of the previously accepted medical procedures that are now considered barbaric and unsuccessful. I can't help but think we will someday look back at many of today's common practices with the same sentiment. Unfortunately, the patient is usually the last to find out that many of these methods are, in fact, dangerous, often at the

---

[3] Obukhanych, Tetyana, PHD. "Vaccine Illusion, How Vaccination Compromises Our Natural Immunity and What We Can Do to Regain Our Health." Amazon Digital Services LLC. February 17, 2012.

expense of their own health and well-being, and many times even their own life. As the saying goes: *"We don't know what we don't know."*

There is a vested interest in upholding vaccine safety, effectiveness, and necessity. The business of vaccines is the major source of profits for the world's largest pharmaceutical corporations. The 'vaccine machine' which is run by Big Pharma is estimated to generate $18 billion by 2020. The flu shot sector alone will generate over 3.8 billion in profits by the end of 2019. An article by Andrea Billups entitled, "How Much Revenue Do Vaccines Generate?" demonstrates that since 1986 vaccines have generated billions of dollars in revenue for drug companies and that "costs paid by the federal government—which purchases half of all the vaccines for the nation's children—have risen 15-fold."[4] Annual immunization costs have grown from $100 per child in 1986 to $2,192 per child in 2015, citing data from the Centers for Disease Control and Prevention.

What is further concerning is that pharmaceutical corporations are financially intertwined with medical universities, hospitals, the Center for Disease Control (CDC), the news, and media outlets. They have infiltrated all of the government agencies that approve and mandate vaccines. The agency's that are supposed to remain objective and defend the interests of the people are failing to do their job. It's a classic case of the fox guarding the hen house. With not much effort, one can easily discover that pharmaceutical companies commonly fund political campaigns, often spending more money than those lobbying for oil and gas. A recent report stated that the pharmaceutical industry is holding up to its title as the top

---

[4] Billups, Andrea. "How Much Revenue do Vaccines Generate?" Newsmax.com. June 27, 2015.

lobbying force in Washington. In 2019, drugmakers had spent more than $129 million through September which was slightly down from nearly $133 million the year prior, but still far more than any other industry.[5]

What should raise more red flags is that vaccines are the only drugs mandated by government and protected from all financial liability. Vaccine manufacturers were quite unhappy that they were being sued for adverse reactions from vaccines and consequently, suffering financially. The vaccine manufacturers threatened to stop all research into new vaccines. As a result, in 1986, Congress passed The National Childhood Injury Act which states that vaccine manufacturers could no longer be sued for injury or vaccine related death. All financial liability was removed from the vaccine manufacturers. This opened the door for further vaccine research and new vaccine production. To admit that the science behind vaccinations is outdated and flawed does not help the vaccine machine. This multi-billion-dollar industry has no incentive to admitting negligence.

In 1986, Congress also appointed the US Department of Health and Human Services the role of monitoring vaccine adverse events and injuries. The US Departments of Health and Human Services were ordered to report to various agencies every three years to ensure vaccines were safe and effective. In over thirty-three years, they have failed to do so. On October 12, 2019, the Informed Consent Action Network (ICAN) filed a lawsuit against The Department of Health and Humans Services. They pleaded guilty for failing to do what they were assigned to do; ensuring that the vaccines added to

[5] Evers-Hillstrom, Karl. "Big Pharma continues to top lobbying spending". October 25,2019. OpenSecrets.org. https://www.opensecrets.org/news/2019/10/big-pharma-continues-to-top-lobbying-spending/

the childhood vaccine schedule are benefiting our children and not harming them.

Prior to 1986, babies received seven different vaccinations. Since then, we have added more vaccines, added booster shots and started administering vaccines right after birth. By the time a baby reaches eighteen months, a fully vaccinated child will receive 38 vaccines for sixteen different diseases. The tough questions that must be asked are: Are these vaccines safe? Are these vaccines improving the health of our children? If vaccines are truly safe, why are the vaccine manufacturers protected from liability?

Consider this: an entire industry is profiting from incorrect, outdated and harmful information. As a society, we must be willing to let go of our old beliefs as more appropriate concepts are discovered and understood. Throughout history, we have witnessed many 'tipping points' where world trends seemed to magically change. My dream is that we soon reach one of those tipping points where we get back to the basics and change the horrifying direction our country's health is going toward. My heart goes out to those who have been injured and will be injured as we continue in this downward spiral. I do, however, feel hopeful as there are many tools to help those who are injured, and we currently still hold the power to fight for our medical rights.

Medical freedom is eroding, and unfortunately, Big Pharma has no intention of changing that. But I do believe that as more people become educated, more will be willing to fight for the ability to maintain our medical freedom.

"Of all the anti-social vested interests, the worst is the vested interest in ill-health." - George Shaw

Chapter 3

Protecting the Unborn

The infant's immune system starts to develop by the 5th week of pregnancy and the thymus is open for business...it invites the stem cells to learn to become T-cells and they direct the immune response post birth. The (TH1) arm of the immune system (infection fighting arm) begins in utero but is suppressed in utero so baby doesn't attack mom and mom doesn't attack baby.

The infant's immune balance is influenced by the mother's lifestyle: how she eats, exposure to heavy metals from vaccinations, medications, smoking, prescription and over-the-counter drugs, and alcohol. All of these variables have a direct effect on the baby's immune system and neurological development.

For years, it was common knowledge that you never gave a pregnant mother a vaccine or medication that contained mercury or aluminum. The babies under-developed brain and nervous system are considered vulnerable to injury from toxic exposures. When a pregnant mother gets a vaccine with aluminum or mercury, it can disrupt the delicate balance in the unborn child and lead to neurological problems that show up later as learning problems, ADHD, autism....

In today's world, it is impossible for one to avoid all toxins in the environment. Still, the pregnant mother must try her best to avoid exposing her growing baby to any form of toxic exposures. The fetuses developing brain and body is delicate and must be protected. The placenta provides oxygen and nutrients to the growing baby and removes waste from the baby's blood, but the placenta can only protect the baby to a certain degree. A study led by the Environmental Working Group (EWG) examined the umbilical cord blood of 10 U.S. babies born in 2004. What they found was that there was an average of 200 industrial chemicals and pollutants found in the cord blood. Of the 287 chemicals detected in the umbilical cord blood, 180 were known to cause cancer in humans or animals, 208 were known to cause birth defects or abnormal development in animal tests, and 217 were known to be toxic to the brain and nervous system. EWG senior scientist, Anita Jacobs, stated, "We know the developing fetus is one of the most vulnerable populations, if not the most vulnerable, to environmental exposure. Their organ systems aren't mature, and their detox methods are not in place, so cord blood gives us a good picture of exposure during this most vulnerable time of life...the developing fetus is one of the most vulnerable populations, if not the most vulnerable."[6]

We may not have control over the hundreds of environmental chemicals we are exposed to in our air, water, and food daily; but we do, however, have control over whether we take drugs and medications while pregnant and our overall lifestyle choices. One common practice I find quite disconcerting is the encouragement from OBGYNs for pregnant women to receive the seasonal influenza and DTaP vaccines. These vaccinations, which contain large amounts of aluminum, possibly thimerosal (a form of mercury), and many other chemicals. The package insert that accompanies these

---

[6] Environmental Working Group. "Body Burden: The Pollution in Newborns." EWG.org. July 14, 2005.

immunizations state that they have not been tested for safety on pregnant mothers. The FDA's Influenza Vaccine insert clearly states, "There are, however, no adequate and well-controlled studies in pregnant women." One can assume that they have not been studied in relation to how they affect the development of the unborn baby either.

The flu season from 2009-2010 was the first time in which flu shots were recommended for pregnant women. When analyzing the data reported in VAERS (Vaccine Adverse Event Reporting System), during this flu season miscarriage rates increased from 7 to 128 cases reported. Furthermore, the 2009 H1N1 inactivated-influenza vaccination program contributed to an estimated 1,688 miscarriages and stillbirths among women 17 to 45 years of age. In this same year, my daughter, Dr. Renee Hunter, testified before the CDC on behalf of the Coalition of Organized Women to express concerns about these statistics. During her testimony, she posed the question: Why are these vaccines recommended during pregnancy when there are statistics showing increases of fetal death? The panel members refused to respond to the testimony and seemed uninterested. In attendance was Dr. Marie McCormick, the chair of H1N1 Vaccine Risk Assessment Working Group. She reported that "There have been no adverse events in the pregnant population," blatantly disregarding the reports made to VAERS. Despite the shocking reports and lack of safety studies, the flu shots are recommended every year to pregnant women.

Another vaccine that poses concern is the RhoGAM vaccine, a vaccine for pregnant women who are blood type Rh-negative. This vaccine is generally recommended at three separate times throughout pregnancy and may contain thimerosal (mercury) and/or polysorbate 80, which has caused infertility in mice.[7] Personally, I am Rh-negative and after researching the vaccine, decided against receiving it for four of my five pregnancies. It was the right decision for me, and you will have to choose what the right decision is for yourself. On my website www.ChildhoodShots.com I have provided a helpful article about the Rhogam vaccine. (Under Health Articles: "What is The Rhogam Vaccine?").

I encourage all pregnant women to pull the vaccine manufacturer's vaccine insert called the 'Product Monograph' and review it thoroughly prior to agreeing to any vaccine. Examine the warnings section, adverse reactions section, and toxicology section. Research any information you do not understand so that you are able to make an informed decision. I want you to know that you do have options and once thoroughly researched, you will be equipped to make the right decision for yourself.

Never in the history of humankind have we introduced, via injection, synthetic drugs during pregnancy, vaccinations at birth, and then more vaccinations throughout life. The long-term health consequences of such practices are not yet fully grasped and the ramifications of these methods on future generations are unknown. Unfortunately, unborn children in the US are developing in some very undesirable conditions. If mothers listen to their good-intended, but often ignorant doctors, their babies are presented with a huge disadvantage. As parents, it is our duty and responsibility to protect our children at all cost from things that may cause harm.

---

[7] Gajdova M, Jakubovsky J, Valky J.Delayed effects of neonatal exposure to Tween 80 on female reproductive organs in rats. Food Chem Toxicol. 1993 Mar;31(3):183-90. PMID: 8473002

Chapter 4

The Relationship Between Natural Birth and Immunity

Vaginal birth is very important. Remember, the baby's immune system has been suppressed by "Mother Nature" so the baby and mom don't fight each other. Passing through the birth canal (vaginal delivery) stimulates the Th1 immune system into action. This amazing process is very important to the child's future health. Also, compression of the baby's body while traveling down the birth canal initiates the natural maturation of infant reflexes, allowing proper neural development to take place. This journey through the birth canal is the first stage of natural immunity stimulation. This is one of the reasons why vaginal delivery is important. If a child is born via C-section, they do not have this advantage. When we interfere with the natural process through, synthetic oxytocin, C-sections and formula feeding, we disturb the natural progression, leading to what are known as "diseases of intervention."

As a result, conditions such as allergies, asthma, and diabetes can occur and can set the person up for obesity, autoimmune disease, and even cancer later in life. If the immune system is not allowed to hit important natural milestones, it oftentimes does not get it right later.

Healthier children have a Th1 dominant immune system and life-long immunity because Th1 cells are the infection fighters, especially intracellular viral infections. The "Gold Standard" of public health, as a valid sign of efficacy in vaccinology, is the measurement of a high titer antibody response. Antibodies are only one small part of the entire picture. Antibody titers only reflect exposure and do not represent immunity. Current science knows high antibody levels may be a sign of chronic on-going infection and susceptibility to infection.

For the past hundred years, scientists and doctors have believed that humans develop in a womb that remains sterile and completely isolated from bacteria, fungi, and viruses. Newly emerging research has shown that microorganisms are likely present inside the womb during normal development. These microorganisms slowly and steadily accumulate in the fetus during pregnancy establishing the baby's microbiome in the womb. When a baby is born vaginally, they acquire additional beneficial microbes from the mother's feces which coats their mouth, nose, gastrointestinal tract, and body. These microbes consist of bacteria, fungi, viruses and other organisms unique to the mother's body. The microbe transfer that occurs during vaginal delivery is very beneficial and ideal for the baby as it supports gut and immune system development. A 2007 study entitled "Importance of Microbial Colonization of the Gut in Early Life to the Development of Immunity," concludes that:

"The mammalian gastrointestinal tract harbors a complex microbiota consisting of between 500 and 1000 distinct microbial species. Comparative studies based on the germ-free gut have provided clear evidence that the gut microbiota is instrumental in promoting the development of both the gut and systemic immune system. Early microbial exposure of the gut is thought to dramatically reduce the incidence of inflammatory, autoimmune and atopic diseases, further fueling the scientific viewpoint, that microbial colonization plays an important role in regulating and fine-tuning the immune system throughout life. However, much remains to be elucidated about how commensal bacteria influence the function of cells of both the innate and adaptive immune systems in health and disease."

The study continues:

"This data supports the notion that the composition of gut microbiota in infants can be influenced by the type of infant feeding, and other factors including mode of delivery, gestation age, infant hospitalization, and antibiotic treatment. Delivery by cesarean section, for example, not only prevents the newborn from being exposed to bacteria in the birth canal but also decreases the general bacterial exposure from the mother because of routine antibiotic prophylaxis in cesarean delivery. In comparison with vaginally delivered infants, the gut of the cesarean section-delivered infant has lower numbers of (good bacteria) bifidobacteria and Bacteroides."[8]

Another article by Scientific American called, "Among Trillions of Microbes in the Gut, a Few Are Special," states:

"In 2012 the National Institutes of Health completed the first phase of the Human Microbiome Project, a multimillion-dollar effort to catalogue and understand the microbes that inhabit our bodies. The microbiome varies dramatically from one individual to the next and can change quickly over time in a single individual. The great majority of the microbes live in the gut, particularly the large intestine, which serves as an anaerobic digestion chamber. Scientists are still in the early stages of exploring the gut microbiome, but a burgeoning body of research suggests that the makeup of this complex microbial ecosystem is closely linked with our immune function."[9]

---

[8] Kelly, Denise. King, Timothy. Aminov, Rustam. "Importance of Microbial Colonization of the Gut in Early Life to the Development of Immunity." Mutation Research/Fundamental and Molecular Mechanisms of Mutagenesis. Volume 622, Issue 1-2. September 1, 2007.

[9] Velasquez-Manoff, Moises. "Among of Microbes in the Gut, a Few Are Special." *Scientific American.* March 1st, 2015.

Beneficial bacteria in the body is vital to health and promotes a strong immune system. As previously stated, C-section deliveries prevent the baby from being exposed to these healthy bacteria, leaving them vulnerable to health issues later in life.

C-sections have skyrocketed in the U.S. since the mid- 1970s. In a single generation, the country's C-section rate has increased 500 percent. The World Health Organization suggests that the optimal rate of C-sections lies between 10 and 15 percent. Currently, North America is well above the optimal rate, with 32 percent of all babies delivered by C-section. This means 1 in 3 births result in a C-section. Salimah Walani, the vice president of global programs at March of Dimes states, "The procedure is done when it is not really necessary or indicated. The surgical procedure can do more harm than good for moms and babies."[10] It is speculated that three factors are driving the global rise of C-sections: financial (C-sections are more profitable), legal, and technical. For a mom, electing to have a C-section raises the chance of death by a minimum of 60 percent and greatly increases the risk of life-threatening complication during childbirth. The statistics are equally concerning for the baby as C-sections increase the probability of health issues later in life such as autoimmune diseases and obesity. We are only beginning to understand the lifelong effects of babies born via C-section. The microbial

---

[10] Doucleff, Michelle. "Rate of C-Sections Is Rising at an 'Alarming' Rate, Report Says." NPR, Women & Girls, October 12, 2018.
https://www.npr.org/sections/goatsandsoda/2018/10/12/656198429/rate-of-c-sections-is-rising-at-an-alarming-rate.

transfer from a vaginal birth provides lifelong benefits, but with a C-section this doesn't happen.

If beneficial bacteria are not plentiful, the educational process for the immune system is impaired and can result in unwanted health issues. I find that many expecting mothers are unaware of the immense benefits of a vaginal delivery. It is imperative that we educate mothers on the importance of natural birth and encourage vaginal birth when possible. The development of the gut microbiome must be protected as it is our first line of defense.

Chapter 5

The Development and Feeding of Microbes in Infancy

Breast feeding is the most effective way to encourage healthy immunity and support growth and development the first years of life. Colostrum, the first milk produced, will encourage the Th1 arm and help good microbes and bacteria colonization in the digestive system (the gut). Over 75% of our immune system is in the gut so breast feeding is extremely important to help develop a healthy defense system. Mother will transfer her own immunity to the child via breast milk giving the child a measure of protection the first several months of life.

Children who receive vaccinations on day 1 in the hospital have a very different immune response. Vaccines cause an immune system reaction pushing it in the opposite direction, to the Th2 arm of the immune system, causing an imbalance. Getting the vaccines results in a temporary immunity (by suppression) meaning that susceptibility is deferred, and repeated booster shots will be required for the entire life of the individual."

Breastfeeding (nursing) promotes healthy microbial colonization of the infant's digestive system. The first milk produced by the mother, colostrum, is packed full of various nutrients and antibodies that are not found in formula. Colostrum is a yellow, concentrated milk that is produced in small amounts and performs many vital functions. It creates a tough coating on the baby's stomach and intestines to prevent germs from causing illness, helps prevent low blood sugar in newborns, helps support the liver, and delivers stem cells needed to repair any post birth problems. The colostrum provides everything the brand-new digestive system needs;

packed full of protein, fats, vitamins, and salts to create complete nutrition. It is ideal for supporting the immune system and organs and sets the stage for the rich milk that will follow in days to come.

Breastmilk is a super food. According to Psychology Today:

"Breast milk contains the "perfect combination of proteins, fats, vitamins and carbohydrates" for newborn development. The same study indicates that Infants who are exclusively breast fed for 12 months or longer, have 20-30 percent increased brain growth compared with formula fed infants. The cells in the brain are largely made from a group of long-chained polyunsaturated fatty acids called DHA (docosahexaenoic acid) and A (arachidonic acid) and breast milk is the perfect nutritional support for brain and nervous system development."[11]

Furthermore, an informative article called "The Composition of Breast Milk Over Time: What's in it? And How Does it Change?" further describes:

"During breastfeeding, the suckling creates a vacuum and forces a mixture of breast milk and baby's saliva to go back upstream into the mother's nipple, called, "baby spit backwash". This "retrograde milk flow" from the baby's mouth to the mother's nipple, produces on-demand immune cells for baby! The immune cells, called leukocytes, are then passed back to baby through breast milk, helping baby fight the infection. Although still being studied, this idea of tailored immunity makes sense. A key concept of immunity is the exposure to pathogens. This triggers the immune system to respond and fight back. Breast milk contains millions

[11] Bergland, Christopher. "Breastfeeding Boosts the Brain Development of a Baby." Psychology Today. June 8, 2013.

of live cells. These include immune-boosting white blood cells, as well as stem cells, which may help organs develop and heal." [12]

Ideally, the mother should consume healthy, organic foods to provide the very best milk for her newborn. According to the research conveyed previously in this chapter, there are true advantages seen with breast-fed-only nutrition for the first 12 months of life. I encourage mothers to strive for that 12-month mark, and at that time, if the baby shows interest in foods one can begin the gradual introduction of whole foods. The longer a mother breastfeeds, the better. I breastfed all five of my children for at least the first two years of life and a few beyond. As a baby grows, the gut forms a barrier between the walls of the colon and the blood stream which is referred to as the gut-blood barrier. This barrier forming process can take several months and by introducing food too early, this process can be interrupted.

The use of breast pumps has made life easier for mothers around the world, particularly for those who work. The working mother who takes time to pump her milk so that her child can have the best nutrition deserves a round of applause, however, it must be stated that side effects are rarely mentioned when discussing the use of breast pumps. For one, the continuous use of a breast pump can greatly reduce the amount of milk a mother produces. The mechanism of a latching baby is what stimulates more milk. For those who pump and then store the breast milk, it is shown that freezing or refrigerating the breast milk and then thawing it can cause depletion of nutrients. Other side effects of using breast

---

[12] Family and Co. Nutrition.com. "The Composition of Breast Milk Over Time." February 12, 2019.

pumps include potential nipple and breast tissue damage. I would allow the baby to latch on as often and as much as possible and use the breast pump only when it is absolutely needed.

In some cases, mothers have trouble producing breastmilk. Various contributions can cause trouble in producing milk, such as: hormonal issues, poor newborn latching, not breastfeeding often enough or long enough, being on certain medications and I have even witnessed emotional disturbances contribute to low milk production. Luckily, if milk supply is low there are some great options. In my opinion, donor breast milk is the best alternative in this situation. In most cities you may find online milk banks where breast milk can be either purchased or even donated. I recommend meeting with the mother who is donating milk and ask detailed questions about her lifestyle habits (foods, medications, etc.) to ensure you are getting healthy breast milk for your baby. This can be a Godsend for the mother and infant! My daughter-in-law was having trouble producing breast milk and was able to get some from a mother that ate organically, lived a healthy lifestyle, had a healthy baby and happened to make a lot of extra milk. There are ways to properly store breastmilk, so be sure to do your research and ask the donor mother a lot of questions. Breast milk is far better than any formula one can purchase. It is important to remember that one is not just feeding a hungry baby, but also feeding the brain, the gut, and the gut microbiome.

When your child is ready to start eating solid foods, what you choose to start feeding them matters considerably. Your choices will either promote unhealthy microbes, like yeast and fungi, or the promotion of healthy bacteria. Foods high in sugar and simple carbohydrates may allow unhealthy fungus and yeast to proliferate. I greatly encourage parents to start with organic, green vegetables which are naturally lower in sugar. It is generally a good rule of thumb to add them gradually while observing any skin rashes or diaper rashes which could indicate a sensitivity to that food. The topic is so detailed and vast, I could dedicate a whole book to it! Luckily, there are many resources on the internet with supported research and suggestions on how to introduce foods carefully. I also have many articles on my website discussing how to eat while pregnant and nursing, and ways to support natural immunity. Those articles can be found on www.ChildhoodShots.com (Under the topic: "Raising Kids").

Providing parents don't allow other factors to interfere with normal immune system development, a baby will thrive and grow stronger with each passing week.

"A newborn has only three demands. They are warmth in the arms of its mother, food from her breasts, and security in the knowledge of her presence. Breastfeeding satisfies all three."

Dr. Grantly Dick-Read

Chapter 6

Educating the Army for Strong Defense

Infants get exposed to all bacteria, fungi, viruses, infectious pathogens through their mouth, nose, ears and lungs; these are the natural portal-of-entries into the body. Over time, the Th2 arm of the immune system develops by being exposed multiple times to pathogens as the child lives. Occasionally as children grow, they may also get cuts or wounds or an insect bite on the skin where the immune system is visibly active in the healing process as it swells and responds to the foreign substance injected by the insect.

It is no accident that babies put everything in the mouth. By a few months of age, they start tasting everything and this activity will increase as they begin to teethe. This is the way the internal body gets to know about the environment the baby is living in. When they begin to expose themselves to the many different pathogens in their environment, (mold, fungus, dust, bugs, bacteria from animals…) the immune system (TH1) kicks into action and the process to identify, attack and eliminate the foreign pathogens begins. Millions of times throughout the day, a newborns body is responding to foreign things from its environment. They are often fighting things internally and we are not aware of the amazing combat taking place as they learn about the world around them.

It is common for babies to have runny noses, fevers, swollen glands and body rashes as the immune system filters foreign invaders out through the different excreting portals. They are getting exposed thousands of times daily to this environment and they must learn to adopt and thrive in spite of the environment. This is all part of normal, natural immune development.

These quotes explain much about the intricate design of what God created. The only way our bodies grow and develop is by experiencing life and learning from it. There is no short-cut to healthy immune development. The process of immune development takes time and requires freedom of the child to experience life naturally. Babies crawl on the floor for many months, putting everything they find in their mouths: Dog bones, dust, toys, and sometimes, even bugs. With every new object touched to the mouth, the body is instructed and trained in how to process and proceed. This is how the T-Cells, the infection fighting soldiers of the immune system, will learn about the that baby's environment.

I still remember the taste of the dog Milk-Bones I ate when I was three and will never forget the chocolate covered bumblebees my older brother gave me to eat when I was ten. My younger brother, Billy, unknowingly ate the chocolate covered ants and when he found out what they were, he threw up immediately. He should have tried the bumblebees! Being number seven of eleven children sure provided many exciting experiences.

I encouraged my babies to play in the grass and walk barefoot in the dirt. We puddle-stomped and played in rivers and lakes. I loved to see them in the woods climbing trees, playing in the leaves; catching bugs and frogs. I was never fearful about germs and I let them get dirty. Through raising my five children, I observed that the first seven years of life are filled with various symptoms: colds, fevers (commonly seen with teething), swollen glands, runny noses, coughs, sore throats, skin rashes and sometimes sleeping issues. These normal immune 'exercises' are signs that the body's immune system is working and developing. Many times, it is painful and unpleasant, but it is these exercises that build a major network of immune fighters. I also observed that some of my children seemed to be more sensitive and symptomatic than others.

I view body symptoms not as a sign of something bad, but more so a sign that the body is working. For instance, if you eat a bad piece of fish and you suddenly throw up, are you sick? In this case, is the action of throwing up a good thing or a bad thing? These are signs that the body is working effectively to rid itself of something that is harmful. This is a normal and vital function. If a child eats something that their body doesn't want, it must come out. This may result in vomiting, diarrhea, fevers or rashes (the skin which is the largest organ does a great job at filtering out toxins). These are all ways that the body fights and protects itself by removing dangerous organisms.

I would like to share a true and related story. My son Curtis went out shrimping with his friend on the intercoastal waters of Charleston, SC. After devouring his newly caught, fresh, raw shrimp, he called me to tell me how delicious it was. Mortified, I informed him of the dangers in eating raw shrimp and told him not to take another bite. He reassured me that he was "strong" and "never gets sick", which was usually the case. We all know teenagers: they always know better than their mothers! The next day he was traveling to Michigan to visit family when I got a call saying that he was very ill. He was suffering with green diarrhea, was vomiting, running a fever and felt awful. These are all normal bodily reactions to consuming raw seafood that was obviously tainted with harmful bacteria; more than likely, Salmonella, E. coli, or Vibrio. As soon as he arrived, I provided him with an all-natural product called: Biocidin (formulated by Bio-Botanical Research). Biocidin is a combination of botanical compounds which are naturally anti-viral and anti-bacterial. This product does a great job in supporting the body through times like this. He was encouraged to rest, stay hydrated and within two days he was feeling much better. His body was doing exactly what it was designed to do, fight and eject an invading organism. We decided to support his body with a non-invasive, immune supporting product. I assure you, if we would have taken him to a medical clinic, they would have prescribed an antibiotic (which destroys both harmful and beneficial bacteria). If he had not shown improvements or was having worsening symptoms, we would have explored this option, but my family always views medical interventions as a last resort.

My husband and I took the job of exposing our children to the world seriously. When their bodies functioned as God intended by displaying symptoms, we did not refer to them as 'sick', but instead 'under-the-weather'. I would do my best to comfort my children through this process by preparing nourishing foods for them like chicken soup, teaching them that their body was fighting, and the symptoms would pass soon. Ultimately, there are no short-cuts; we cannot skip the immune exercise drills if we want a strong defensive immune. The immune system must go through boot-camp to develop.

It is astonishing how every childhood disease I contracted as a child is now referred to as "life-threatening and dangerous." Prior to vaccines, these illnesses were called "normal childhood illnesses." When I was growing up, all my siblings contracted the chickenpox, measles, mumps and many other normal childhood illnesses just as every other kid I knew. After a week of fevers and rashes, we were blessed with life-long immunity to those infections that our bodies recovered from. In the 1950s, 450,000 children a year would contract these common illnesses and death rates from them were very low. It was not uncommon to see episodes featuring these childhood illnesses in old television shows like the Brady Bunch. In fact, an episode in 1966 involved the daughter Marcia staying home from school due to the measles. The mother says, *"A slight temperature, a lot of dots and great big smile!"* Marcia then stated, *"If you have to get sick, sure can't beat the measles!"* This old TV program reflected the cavalier way people felt about measles and the trust we once had in the body and immune system.

Today, this generation of parents are paranoid about all of these illnesses we got as children. Our neighbors would call and tell us if they had a child with the chickenpox so that we could go for a visit and get exposed! My mother would have a few of us each year getting the "special treatment" as we processed these illnesses. I remember having the blinds closed in my bedroom to keep the light down while I had the measles because my eyes were sensitive to it. These illnesses prepared us for adulthood!

Chapter 7

The Working Army

There are 3 basic lines of defense: skin, mucosal membrane, tears, urine, fevers & Inflammation and acquired or adaptive immunity. I describe those areas here:

Skin: The largest organ in the body and part of the integumentary system and the first line of defense. It is made up of multiple layers and protects the muscles, bones, ligaments and internal organs. Because it is exposed to the environment, it plays a key role in protecting the body. It is also porous, so it takes in toxins and also excretes toxins. It protects against excessive water loss and helps with temperature regulation. It allows us to feel and also protects Vitamin D synthesis. The immune system excretes toxins through the skin which may result in rashes. (Chickenpox, measles, allergies…) Mucosal membranes include the nostrils, mouth, lips eyelids, ears, genitalia area and the anus. Many are connected to the glands and produce mucus, which is trapping pathogens in the body to prevent further activity of that pathogen. People call this "sickness", but I refer to it as "immune system function."

Fevers and Inflammation: For years, the fever was feared, parents were told to treat the fever with medication to bring it down. Consider this amazing fact: During a 102-degree fever, the body produces interferon which is a class of protein that prevents viral replication and inhibits cancer cells. Interferon: a natural fighter released to do some miraculous jobs in the body to maintain health and balance. At 103 degrees, the body stores all nutrition in the spleen to starve off harmful bacteria. Bacteria have a very shallow variance of temperature they can live in, (again, another Mother Nature fact that is often misunderstood). This may be when the baby refuses to eat and is suffering with nausea and/or diarrhea. The child may feel weak and be fussy but understand that Mother Nature is doing her job to bring them back to balance. Most childhood illnesses that result in fevers last a few days and will resolve without any medical interventions. Next, inflammation: A very important part of immunity, without inflammation, cuts, wounds, sprained joints and infections cannot heal. Inflammation is a part of a complex biological response of vascular tissues in response to some sort of harmful stimuli: damaged cells, bacteria, foreign particles (sliver of wood, bee sting, cuts…) sprained joints etc. It is one of the first responders to injury and best if left alone to do its work. Acute inflammation will be present until the healing process is done. It is an essential part of the innate immunity process.

Acquired (adaptive or specific) immunity: This is not present at birth and must be learned. Also referred to as specific immunity because it tailors its attack to a specific antigen previously encountered. Its hallmarks are its ability to learn, adapt, and remember. This will take 7 – 10 years to develop and requires "wild" exposure to specific viruses and bacteria common with natural childhood illnesses: chickenpox measles, mumps, diphtheria, rubella etc.…It is the end result of the Th1 arm responding appropriately and over time stimulating Th2.

Each level of the immune system has its own specialized soldiers trained to carry out separate missions. These soldiers remain in close communication with the entire body and know what other soldiers are doing in different parts of the body.

They are never off the clock, continually working, even when we are unaware of the battle being waged on our behalf.

Back in the 1980s, a prominent pediatrician named Barton Schmitt coined the term "fever-phobia" to describe the desire of many parents to bring down fevers in their children as quickly as possible. Here we are in 2019 and fever-phobia is still alive and well. The fever, a vital response initiated by the immune system, serves many important functions. One of those functions is to kill off harmful bacteria. As stated in the beginning of this chapter, bacteria are unable to live in certain temperatures. The body innately knows this and heats up to quickly kill off harmful bacteria. Many physicians are now acknowledging the benefits of the fever and are no longer recommending fever reducers unless the fever reaches 104 degrees. In many other countries, fever reducers are administered only if hospitalized and only when the fever reaches 104 degrees. I was pleased to discover that the American Academy of Pediatrics is no longer recommending reducing fevers. (Took them long enough!) They acknowledge that a fever can help your child's body fight off infection, allowing a fever to run its course may reduce the length and severity of such illnesses as colds and flu.

A study published in the Journal of Allergy and Clinical Immunology found that children who ran a fever during their first year were less likely to develop allergies later in childhood than children who did not have a fever.[13] Unfortunately, many allopathic doctors are still promoting the use of fever reducing medications and often recommend a cocktail of drugs to overcome symptoms. This stands in the way of the body's natural immune process; preventing it from learning and

---

[13] Hurt, Avery. "Benefits of Having a Fever". Parents.
https://www.parents.com/baby/health/fever/what-to-do-when-your-baby-has-a-fever/.

growing stronger. In addition to this, common fever reducing medication such as Tylenol contain Acetaminophen, a compound well known for causing liver failure. To inform yourself of the long list of adverse effects of Acetaminophen an article can be found on my website www.ChildhoodShots.com.

All parents should be made aware of the many natural methods to help reduce fevers if needed. Instead of having fever phobia, one should make themselves experts on not only the functions of a fever, but natural tools to help ease a fever and signs that intervention is needed. Most parents are concerned with the thought of their child having a febrile seizure. It should be mentioned that although quite frightening, the febrile seizure is usually harmless and typically does not indicate a serious health problem. I have found that febrile seizures usually occur due to dehydration in response to a fever. There are many great tips online that ensure your child stays hydrated during illness.

Other symptoms such as runny noses and other classic cold symptoms are just indications that the body is successfully eliminating and detoxing. The body works hard to expel toxics in this natural process, but we are programmed to view this as "sickness". Rather than medicating to reduce these symptoms, I focus on assisting the body. That is what natural health is all about.

Immunologist, Tetyana Obukhanych, PhD frequently discusses the role of nutrition and in particular the role of Vitamin C and D in providing protection for ourselves from various viruses. Vitamin C and D are very important to maintaining our defenses, especially in the autumn and winter months when we are not frequently absorbing the sunlight. Her natural approach focuses on preventing illnesses by supporting immune function and maintaining a natural state of preparedness. Both her and Dr. Marini concur that it is best to get "wild" infections, allowing the body to respond normally and in doing so, develop natural life-long immunity. They also both agree that building the immune system can be a 7 to 10 year process. Immune boosts then happen as we go through life and are exposed to different microorganisms. Unfortunately, immunology is not perceived this way by the medical community because immunologists don't study the immune system. They study vaccinology.

If you find your child seems to have a lot of health challenges, it is wise to take a closer look at what they are eating. Nowadays it is not uncommon for children to have sensitivities to wheat, dairy, soy, food coloring and food additives. My oldest son was very sensitive to dairy. Although we didn't consume milk at home, I found that if he drank some at a friend's or relative's house he would come home with a runny nose, swollen glands and sometimes even a fever. Thankfully, we were able to correlate his symptoms with an intolerance to dairy early-on and greatly limited his consumption. For some children symptoms of food intolerance can present as chronic ear infections, digestive issues or even behavioral disturbances. In some cases, I have witnessed health issues occur in children whom were having trouble adapting to family and life changes. Taking a step back to assess the child's emotional status can be beneficial, as well.

The human body and the innate wisdom within all of us is truly remarkable. I find that supporting this normal immune process is often more about "what not to do". Many of us, due to the way we were raised, are programmed to interfere with the natural bodily processes and stop symptoms. Mothers and fathers need to be involved in healthcare decisions for the family together. As research and understanding is gained, it becomes easier to make sound, fearless decisions when faced with a crisis.

"If it doesn't challenge you, it doesn't change you." - Fred Devito

Chapter 8

The Gut War Zone

Nothing in the human body gets strengthened by avoidance, only by overcoming challenges. As parents, we need to understand the profound power that is part of our God-given ability to fight illnesses and diseases. The focus should be on ways to support natural immune system development and focusing on how to eliminate the toxic chemical burdens that all cause immune system dysregulations.

True lasting health is achieved when the immune system and the nervous system are fully engaged with one another; a beautiful dance that keeps the body in balance. This foundational philosophy of health is based on having the utmost respect for the human body and the innate wisdom within. Innate wisdom always does what is best for the body, whether we understand it or not.

What many people are unaware of is that a huge portion of the immune system resides in GI tract. Our gut is home to a very large number of microbes referred to as the gut microbiota. As we grow, the microbiota shapes the development of our immune system, and the immune system shapes the composition of the microbiota. Our body has a symbiotic relationship with these microbes. These microbes provide essential health benefits to us, and moreover it has become obvious that changes to these microbes can cause immune dysregulation.

Interferences to these beneficial gut microbes must be avoided if one wants to promote a healthy body and immune system. The number one assault on an infant's microbiota is prescribed oral antibiotics within the first years of life. Antibiotics, although lifesaving in many instances, were not designed to be given for every minor infection. The overprescribing of antibiotics has long-since been a mainstream topic of discussion. Not only does overprescribing disrupt the delicate balance of microbes in the GI tract, but also leads to drug resistant strains of bacteria. Antibiotics are not selective when killing bacteria; they kill both the harmful and beneficial bacteria. The discoverer of penicillin, Alexander Fleming, revealed that the nasal mucus (running nose) created when a person suffers from a cold has an inhibitory effect on bacteria. That sounds like a smart immune system to me!

These changes in the gut microbiota not only affect the immune system, but also several other effect important factors. The link between the gut microbiota and how fat is handled and distributed is discussed in a recent study, "The Association Between Antibiotics in the First Year of Life and Child Growth Trajectory". The study concluded that, "At this time, studies have shown that the make-up of the gut microbiota varies between overweight and normal weight individuals, and that changes in weight are associated with changes in the gut microbiota." [14] Obesity in children is a growing concern for both parents and physicians. Currently, one in three kids are overweight. The prevalence of obesity in children has more than tripled from 1971 to 2011. We know that diet, screen time and lack of exercise play a role, as well.

[14] Rhee, Kyung E. and Dawson-Hahn, Elizabeth E. "The Association Between Antibiotics in the First Year of Life and Child Growth Trajectory." *BMC Pediatrics.* January 16, 2019.

When antibiotics are taken and the beneficial bacteria is killed, this can lead to a bacterial imbalance in the gut called dysbiosis. In dysbiosis, the healthy bacteria are killed allowing unhealthy bacteria to flourish and wreak havoc. This in turn causes more symptoms, leading to more antibiotics which causes more dysbiosis. This creates a vicious cycle of further antibiotic treatment. Permanent loss of beneficial bacteria can occur which can lead to life-long *"diseases of intervention"*, which is a term Dr. Marini used to describe the consequences.

Symptoms of dysbiosis are frequent gas or bloating, abdominal cramping, diarrhea, constipation with mucus in the stool, food allergies, leaky gut syndrome, indigestion, Irritable bowel syndrome (IBS), colitis and even colon cancer. The article, "Importance of Microbial Colonization of the Gut in Early Life to the Development of Immunity" notes: "The inter-relationships between the microbiota and the host are clearly important in relation to health and imbalance between these systems appears to drive a wide range of mucosal and systemic immune-mediated disorders, including inflammatory bowel diseases, autoimmune and allergic conditions."[15] We also know that this imbalance in the gut affects the brain leading to neurological development, ADHD/ADD, depression, anxiety and obesity, fungal imbalances throughout the body, leaky gut and later in life, dementia, forgetfulness, brain fog and more.

Modern medicine has turned the natural process of pregnancy and delivery into a huge business. Pregnancy and delivery are treated like an "illness" requiring invasive procedures that are

---

[15] Velasquez-Manoff, Moises. "Among of Microbes in the Gut, a Few Are Special." *Scientific American.* March 1st, 2015.

far from the natural process designed by God. Standard blood work on pregnant women will test for the presence of group Strep B+ (GBS) in the mother. The bacteria that causes GBS normally lives in the intestines, vagina, or rectum and approximately 25% of all healthy women carry GBS bacteria with no symptoms. If the mother tests positive and there is a chance that the child could be exposed while in the birth canal, it is hospital policy that the mother is treated with an IV of antibiotics while in labor for a few hours.

However, this blood work was never performed when I was having my children. I was shocked to learn how many OBGYNs are now ordering the IV and antibiotics as standard procedure. These antibiotics do affect the infant and set the stage for gut microbiota imbalances. If antibiotics are used during labor, there is a good chance it will be present in the breast milk, as well. There are studies showing that almost any drug that's present in your blood will transfer into the breast milk to some degree. Although it may be at low levels, your baby is very small, and the long-term effects are not well understood. It is always better to be safe than sorry. As with all medical interventions, I recommend one does their research, asks their provider questions, reads the drug package inserts, and makes informed decisions. It is good practice to check with the hospital or birthing center to ask what their current policies are. One of the advantages to having a home birth is the ability to avoid many of these unwanted procedures.

"It's easier to fool people than to convince them that they have been fooled."   *-Mark Twain*

Chapter 9

The Big-Pharma-Pseudo-god

According to the Merriam-Webster Dictionary, a ***vaccine is a preparation of killed microorganisms, living attenuated organisms, or living fully virulent organisms that is administered to produce or artificially increase immunity to a particular disease.*** In my opinion this definition is overly simplified and misleading. This general description does not even come close to describing what happens when a vaccine is injected. This simplified definition not only defends the procedure but implies that the vaccine is safe and leads to improved immunity.

As discussed in previous chapters, our understanding of the human body is constantly changing as new science and discoveries emerge. We know very little about the complex immune system and yet all caution is cast aside when it comes to the practice of vaccines. Just in 2008, the discovery of the Interstitium (discussed in depth in chapter 2) provided much information regarding how injected medications and vaccinations circulate the body. This open fluid-filled highway explains how every organ in the body could be introduced to the vaccine, causing an unnatural exposure and reaction. Although the Interstitium is not fully understood, we do know that it drains into the lymphatic system and may explain why some tumors metastasize rapidly once they reach the fluid-filled space. One must wonder, what else travels this fluid-filled highway? When a vaccine is injected deep into the muscle, does it get absorbed by this highway system and travel to other areas of the body? This would explain why vaccines could cause injury in locations far from the injection site (lungs, digestive tract and the brain, to name a few). This is further concerning when we look at the vaccine ingredients and recognize that many of them break down the natural barriers protecting the brain and organs.

Let's reexamine the definition of a vaccination, but this time I will add in key missing information to give a more accurate depiction. A vaccine is **a preparation** (artificially bioengineered viruses, thousands of lab-produced bacteria; developed using body fluids and decomposing organ tissues from sick or decomposing animals, insects, eggs, and aborted fetal tissue) **of killed microorganisms, living attenuated organisms, or fully living virulent organisms** (not found in nature, combined and dangerous, to include preservatives; phenol, 2-phenoxyethanol and thimerosal, germ-killing additives; antibiotics, polysorbate 80 and thimerosal, stabilizers and immune-boosting adjuvants; aluminum, thimerosal and hundreds more), **that is administered** (via deep muscle injection, not only affecting the immune system, but exposing the whole integrated human body: the brain, all organs, tissue, and glands, including the Interstitium), **to produce** (hypothetical and unpredictable) **or artificially increase** (always artificially increasing an immune response by irritation, which is unpredictable, varies and can lead to autoimmune diseases and altered DNA causing genetic mutations) **immunity to a particular disease** (exposure to many different diseases at one time and an immune reaction to everything in the vaccine, not just the viruses, but to all ingredients, including peanuts, dairy, wheat and egg products that are used as adjuvants in vaccines, resulting in food allergies and more).

On February 22, 2011, in the Bruesewitz v. Wyeth LLC case, the Supreme Court ruled vaccines as "unavoidably unsafe." If they are unsafe, then why are they mandated for every child? Every man-made compound, drug or medical procedure has the potential to harm and kill. In many occasions, adverse vaccine reactions are passed off as normal and ignored by doctors. Parents are told that these reactions to vaccines are expected. Unfortunately, the parents often trust the doctor and the child continues to receive vaccinations. If the child dies, or is severely injured, the doctor nor the vaccine company is held liable. The burden of proof falls on the parents to prove their child was injured from the vaccines. There is no pre-testing to evaluate what a child may be sensitive or allergic to. There is ongoing research evaluating how vaccine-induced immune responses and vaccine-related adverse events may be genetically determined. There is strong evidence that suggests that if a family member had a strong reaction to a vaccine, then the child may have a predisposition to injury, as well.

Dr. Gregory Poland, Professor of medicine, founder and leader of Mayo Clinic's Vaccine Research Group, and the world's most admired thinker in modern vaccinology. Dr. Poland is on record stating: "The Measles vaccine is simply a dud, failing to give the protection they think they've acquired. This leads to a paradoxical situation whereby measles in highly immunized societies occurs primarily among those who are immunized."[16] The Mayo Clinic has been trying to determine as to how genetics is affected by the measles vaccine and Dr.

---

[6] Solomon, Lawrence. "I'm No Anti-Vaxxer, But the Measles Vaccine Can't Prevent Outbreaks." *Financial Post.* June 4, 2014.

Poland says: "This may answer many of the deep-seated questions that plague vaccinology... why patients respond so differently to identical vaccines and how to minimize the side effects to vaccination," and how, furthermore, "up to 10 percent of recipients fail to respond to the first dose of the measles vaccine, while another 10 percent generate extremely high levels of measles antibodies. The remaining 80 percent fall somewhere in the middle..." says Dr. Poland: "In no other field of medicine do we do exactly the same thing to everyone—and we do it everywhere in the world."[17] Dr. Poland and I would not agree on much since he is one of the harshest most outspoken critics of anti-vaxxers, but we do agree that vaccines are NOT safe as a one size fits all approach.

What I call the "Big-Pharma-Pseudo-god" wants our trust and unyielding loyalty. It hungers for our faith in it and the "one-size-fits-all" magical vaccines. It tries to make us view our own God-created innate intelligence that formed us from the beginning as flawed. Big-Pharma-pseudo-god demands you deny what you think or feel, do not question and do not try to do anything different because you will harm the flock (herd immunity). The Big-Pharma-Pseudo-god says that vaccines are safe for everyone regardless of genetics, age, weight or health. Furthermore, this false god claims vaccines are so powerful, magical, and failsafe that you can get injected with dozens at one time. But these claims are simply not true. The Big-Pharma-Pseudo-god is indoctrinating us into its flawed dogma of vaccination. Indoctrination closes the mind. It aims to instill in people a set of beliefs that align with a promoted ideology. Indoctrination is often distinguished from education by the fact that the indoctrinated person is expected to not question or critically examine the doctrine they have learned.

---

[17] Mayo Clinic. "Decoding Vaccination: Researchers Reveal Genetic Underpinnings of Response to Measles Vaccine." September 23, 2011.

The potential dangers of taking certain medicines together, is well understood. Pharmacists are very careful to look for drug interactions while dispensing medications. Furthermore, we are just now starting to fully understand how genetics alter one's ability to process drugs and toxins. And yet, vaccines are the Golden Calf that defy all science and medical rationale and our children are given many vaccines at the same time—during the most vulnerable moments of their lives. At well-baby visits, a child will receive up to five injections with nine to thirteen different diseases, in combinational "cocktails"; never tested for safety—all in 60 seconds! Defying all science, these vaccines are deemed perfectly safe, effective and necessary because the Big-Pharma-Pseudo-god says they are.

There is a widely accepted belief that doctors are experts on vaccines and most would assume that doctors receive the best instruction and training into the science of vaccines. Unfortunately, this is not the case. Larry Palevsky, MD, a board-certified pediatrician has this to say about his training in vaccines: "When I went through medical school, I was taught that vaccines were completely safe and completely effective, and I had no reason to believe otherwise. All the information that I was taught was pretty standard in all the medical schools and the teachings and scientific literature throughout the country. I had no reason to disbelieve it. Over the years, I kept practicing medicine and using vaccines and thinking that my approach to vaccines was completely onboard with everything else I was taught. But more and more, I kept seeing that my experience of the world, my experiences in using and reading about vaccines, and hearing what parents were saying about vaccines were very different from what I was taught in medical school and my residency training. It became clearer to me as I read the research, listened to more and more parents, and found other practitioners who also shared the same concern that vaccines had not been completely proven safe or even completely effective, based on the literature that we have today. It also came to my attention that there were ingredients in there that were not properly tested, that the comparison groups were not appropriately set up, and that conclusions made about vaccine safety and efficacy just did not fit the scientific standards that I was trained to uphold in my medical school training."[18] I have found that most doctors are not able to answer basic questions about vaccine ingredients and become quite offended when presented with information contrary to what they were taught in school. Most doctors when presented with questions about aluminum (or another ingredient) amounts in vaccines will revert to fear-mongering tactics about the dangers of the life-threatening diseases. Mothers have reported to me that their doctor responded with, "Don't you be one of those internet mothers who believe all of the anti-vaccine misinformation." Parents are designed with built-in intuition and know their child better than anyone, especially better than the doctor, who has only met the child a few times. It is that God-given intuition that is often undermined by the well-baby visit. A mother (and father's) instincts are amazing. Trust those instincts. They can tell you what to do long before your intellect figures it out.

Fact, doctors and nurses only get ½ day training on vaccines while in school for the purpose of passing their board exams. This has been admitted by hundreds of doctors and nurses.

---

[18] Mercola, Joseph. "Vaccination: The Neurological Poison So Common Your Doctor Probably Pushes It". April 11, 2012.
https://articles.mercola.com/sites/articles/archive/2012/04/11/vaccination-impact-on-childrens-health.aspx

Most do not even know common vaccine ingredients and how they are circulated around the body, absorbed in our organs and tissues.

I encourage parents to just learn a few good facts about ingredients. Aluminum is now in all of the vaccines in huge amounts. No studies have been done on aluminum in the vaccines and yet, doctors will say that vaccines are completely tested and safe. This is not true and they doctor who claims this is dangerous and should be avoided!

Again, many conscientious parents are looking at food labels, buying organic veggies, grass fed beef and free-range chickens. They drink filtered water and watch what their children eat. The research car seats and baby toys to insure they are not toxic and yet, they do not consider what is being injected into their brand-new infants the day they are born and multiple times the first years of life. This must stop. We have already injured two previous generations but this current generation is getting a toxic dump too large to measure.

Social changes take time but once the problem is discovered, we must do what we can to protect our own children and our own communities. Many people are giving up. They believe the problems facing this country are too vast and imbedded in our society to the point of no return. I am a Christian and understand what is predicted in the biblical book of Revelation. I still believe in the mercy and grace of God and therefore, I believe we must do what we can in our local communities. Our children and grandchildren are the beneficiaries of our neglect and our self-absorption. I now acknowledge that even though I home educated my children, I neglected to teach them about their civic duties and the importance of voting locally! I know my generation has failed to protect what we had and as a senior citizen, we do not have the luxury of retiring and just doing what makes us happy!

Post COVID, I think thousands are waking up and acknowledging that we are overrun with fraud and deception in all areas of government. With production of movies like, 2000 Mules, released on May 02, 2022 directed by Dinesh D'Souza, Debbie D'Souza and Bruce Schooley and the book and movie by Robert Kennedy Jr. called, The Real Anthony Fauci: Bill Gates, Big Pharma, and the Global War on Democracy and Public Health, we are able to see the extent of corruption and control being pushed on America and around the world. I believe our elections are rigged and the evil powers that occupy every department and office are feeling the public outcry and pressure. They are running scared and will do what they can to keep us paralyzed in fear. We must expose and eliminate the fraud in our elections, in our schools, in our medical system and in our media.

Do not give up! Our hope and peace come from God who tells us in the book of Ecclesiastes, chapter 3 verses 1-8, there are 28 seasons mentioned in life. It says, "For everything there is a season, a time for every activity under heaven." It does not ever say there is a time to give up! It encourages us to believe that God is working even though we don't see it or feel it. God is working with people like me and you daily to fulfill our purposes and destiny here on Earth.

"It is hard to imagine a more stupid or more dangerous way of making decisions than by putting those decisions in the hands of people who pay no price for being wrong." Thomas Sowell

Chapter 10

The Corruption of Vaccine Research

In this Country we have a medical monopoly that conducts itself more like a medical mafia. My dear friend and mentor, Dr. Tetyana Obukhanych was a traditionally trained Immunologist. Her transition from the laboratory into the world of debate was not easy. She walked away from a secure and respected position because she could no longer be part of the false narrative. I had the privilege of traveling and speaking with her several times. At our speaking engagements, I would present on the dangers of vaccines and she would teach about the role of good nutrition in supporting natural immunity. In her eBook, she gives her opinion of the vaccine program: "It is not immunity that we gain via vaccination but a puny surrogate of immunity. For this reason, vaccination at its core is neither a safe nor an effective method of disease prevention."[19]

When I asked her why the universities never study the dangers of vaccines, she said, "If the committees at the National Institutes of Health (NIH) have decided that it is politically incorrect to study vaccine injuries, then they will turn down

---

[9] Obukhanych, Tetyana, PHD. "Vaccine Illusion, How Vaccination Compromises Our Natural Immunity and What We Can Do to Regain Our Health." Amazon Digital Services LC. February 17, 2012.

any grant application that proposes to do that, no matter how well scientifically justified." There is no money in researching the dangers of vaccines. The NIH has control over what the universities study, research and investigate. Any study contrary to their narrative is ignored or discredited.

The medical mafia has their minions who work hard to stack up the vaccine schedule and create more profit for the vaccine manufacturers. In return they are protected and rewarded financially. Paul Offit, an infectious disease doctor at the Children's Hospital in Philadelphia, is a major spokesperson for the vaccine machine. He owned the patent on a Rotavirus vaccine (for diarrhea in 3rd world countries) called RotaShield. He received $350,000 from Merck to develop the vaccine in 1998 while he was a sitting member of the Vaccine Advisory Board. He voted for the RotaShield to be included in the vaccine program. Due to inadequate testing, the vaccine was pulled off the market six months later because children were dying from intussusception of the colon (a condition in which one segment of intestine "telescopes" inside of another, causing intestinal blockage). Paul suffered no consequences whatsoever. Apparently, conflict of interest is okay when it comes to vaccines. Dr. Offit also previously sat on the CDC's Advisory Committee on Immunization Practices, is a listed inventor on a cluster of vaccine patents in the US and in Europe and currently holds a chair with the IOM (Institute of Medicine) for 1.5 million dollars. This is just one example of the mass corruption happening behind the scenes. This is also an example of why we are in trouble with the mandated vaccine program, why dangers of vaccines are not studied and why natural immunity is ignored.

When research demonstrating the dangerous side of vaccinations is published, the medical mafia attacks the doctors personally seeking to discredit them, professionally terminated or even have their medical licenses revoked. Dr. W. John Martin's story provides a prime example of the repercussions that ensue when speaking out against the medical mafia. Dr. Martin received his medical training in Australia, was the chief of the Immunology/Molecular Pathology Unit at the LAC/USC (University of California) Medical Center as well as a professor of pathology at the USC School of Medicine. In the US, he was the former director of the Vital Oncology Branch of the FDA's Bureau of Biologics which is the principal agency in charge of testing human vaccines. Dr. Martin got fired from the FDA for exposing that the polio vaccines were contaminated with the cytomegalovirus (a virus related to herpes that causes cold sores). I met Dr. Martin in 2005 at a conference and interviewed him on what transpired. Dr. Martin shared with me that when he discovered the cytomegalovirus in the polio vaccines, which were developed on the kidneys of Green African monkeys, he reported it to the FDA immediately. He also identified another virus he labeled the "stealth virus" due to its ability to hide from the immune system and cause chronic inflammation in the brain, organs, and joints. He reported these findings to the FDA Viral Oncology Branch several times. His findings were ignored, and he was forbidden from publishing his findings or making them public. He decided to publish his findings anyway as he was fed up with their desire to cover up this information. As a result, he was relieved of his position and removed from the lab. The FDA worked tirelessly to discredit him and continue to harass him to this day, accusing him of fraud. Dr. Martin stated, "The Food and Drug Administration (FDA) recognized the probable contamination of some polio vaccines in African monkey studies performed in 1972. Yet, public health officials chose to not publicly disclose these studies. It would have raised questions regarding the basic decision to use monkey kidney cells to produce live polio vaccines. Acknowledging this error would also expose the potential origin of HIV, the AIDS virus, from the experimental testing of contaminated polio vaccines in Africa." He has spent the last several years conducting research for a non-profit charity specializing in the study of viruses causing mental illness.

Judy A Mikovits, PhD, has an equally devastating story. Dr. Mikovits had a well-established history working with the National Cancer Institute. Her research focused on immunotherapy. In 2009, while working on autism and related neurological diseases, she found that many of the subjects of the study had motor-neuron diseases, cancer and chronic fatigue syndrome. It was her suspicion that these symptoms were caused by a virus. Through her research, she was able to isolate the virus and conclude that it came from mice. She states, "It looked like a virus, it smelled like a virus, a retrovirus, because those are the types of viruses that disrupt the immune system. And several other investigators back in the 90s had actually isolated retroviruses from these people but the government called them 'contaminants,' that they weren't real and that they didn't have anything to do with the disease. Well, we isolated a new family of viruses that were called xenotropic murine leukemia virus-related virus. So, these viruses were murine leukemia viruses, mouse viruses. So, spin forward two years, our paper published in one of the best scientific journals in the world in Science, October 8th, 2009. Usually that makes one's career, in my case it ended my life as a scientist as I knew it." It wasn't until two years after her research was published that another paper made the connection between this new virus and vaccines. In 2011, a paper written for a journal called Frontiers in Microbiology concluded that the most likely way that these murine leukemia viruses entered humans was through vaccines. Once these implications from the paper became clear, her life as she knew it changed. Dr. Mikovits states, "I was fired, jailed without cause, without hearing, without any civil rights at all, just drug out of my house in shackles one day. On November 18th, 2011, I refused to denounce the data, I refused to say it was a mistake. We have the data. I showed the data. I showed all of the data, and I just refused. They basically said, 'tell everybody you made it all up and you can go home, and if you don't, we'll destroy you.' And they did." There are now testing protocols to detect retroviruses based on Dr. Mikovits' research. This testing protocol is worth millions of dollars and is being managed by Big Pharma. [20]

Another example of how vaccine failures are swept under the rug is what is referred to as the Cutter Incident. In 1955, more than 200,000 children received the polio vaccine, in which the process of inactivating the live virus was defective. Within days, there were 40,000 cases of polio directly caused by the vaccine. This resulted in 200 children with varying degrees of paralysis and killed at least 10 children.[21] This incident was quickly covered up and the new oral sugar cube was put in its place.

Breaking News: In December 2-3, 2019, the Global Vaccine Safety summit with the World Health Organization (WHO) admitted that there are not sufficient safety programs in place to monitor post-marketing vaccines. Several comments are

---

[20] Enos, Richard. "Researcher Jailed After Uncovering Deadly Virus Delivered Through Human Vaccines". Alternative News. Collective Evolution. November 6,2018. https://www.collective-evolution.com/2018/11/06/researcher-jailed-after-uncovering-deadly-virus-delivered-through-human-vaccines/?fbclid=IwAR0Ouj1OoHWq_T0U_ixwQLqpqDekz1sUUncDCWJ3k7flungZpWtuJEZqXF8.

[21] Fitzpatrick, Michael. "The Cutter Incident: How America's First Polio Vaccine Led to a Growing Vaccine Crisis". J R Soc Med. 2006 Mar; 99(3): 156.

worth noting here. They stated that medical doctors and nurses, "Are, *lucky to get a half day of training in school.*" Another member admitted that they do not understand how the "adjuvants" work in the body and that all vaccines are not effective without these adjuvants. Another member admitted that the Influenza vaccine given to pregnant women is "off label" and no studies are done with the pregnant population! One doctor tracking the trends around the world said that the anti-vaccine movement is growing 500% compared to the pro-vaccine camp. They also show concern that primary physicians are losing confidence and faith in the vaccine program.

The W.H.O. illustrated how incompetent they are in regards to safety and up-to-date studies. The video footage is available on YouTube: **The Highwire with Del Bigtree, <u>W.H.O. is lying to Who?</u>** (Episode 145). This is a two-hour production and about 40 minutes into this video, it gets really good! Please watch and share with everyone before it is removed!

The truth is coming out and no one can deny that the safety studies have not been done, post surveillance is not happening and the people running this program are completely incompetent. These lies about unsafe vaccines trickles right down to our own government, the CDC, the FDA, the AAP and to the doctors who are pushing vaccines and continue to defend them as safe and effective. It is as though whatever is in the vile labeled, "Vaccine", it is "holy water" and can do no harm and defies all science and logic.

Even though the vaccine manufactures spend millions on promotion and advertising, financially support candidates running for office and own and control all of the news media outlets, they are losing ground fast.

Physicians are losing faith in the system because parents are questioning them about the safety concerns and they are not equipped to defend the vaccines. Parents of vaccine injured children are showing up by the thousands on capitol steps, protesting the removal of our "religious" rights and shouting for medical freedom to choose the form of healthcare they want for their families. The un-vaccinated children are being wrongly blamed for outbreaks and discriminated against. Their parents are told that they are putting the immune compromised in danger and are selfish.

After 40 years on the frontline of this battle, I am starting to feel like the trend is turning in our favor. I used to know everyone personally who was fighting and educating on the dangers of vaccines. Not so anymore! Now, there are thousands of medical doctors, nurses, pediatricians, PhDs, chiropractors, midwives, homeopaths, naturopaths, nutritionists, herbalists, radio hosts, freedom-fighting groups, autism groups, medical freedom-fighters, radio talk show hosts and Podcast hosts, who are sounding the alarm loud and clear across the globe.

The mama bears have been woken and prodded, their baby bears have been injured and they are relentlessly on the war-path. Fathers are now joining in the fight as they witnessed their young boys quietly drifting away into the autism abyss. Leaders with injured children are speaking out, the gloves are on and the fight is in full-force. This movement will not be stopped and will not go away, and I could not be any prouder!

As we watch the whole vaccine program come unraveled, we all need to know how to promote health so that we can live and enjoy our lives.

We need to hold our leaders accountable. We also need to revoke the vaccine bill of 1986, US Court of Federal Claims, no-fault system, protecting the vaccine manufactures from all financial liability. More on that topic later!

10-24-2022 Update
I am now on Telegram, MeWe, Instagram, Rumble, Gab and other platforms where our speech is not censored. (Search for my name and join channels) Facebook has been censoring all my information and Youtube has removed dozens of live lectures, radio interviews and many video interviews that were archived there for over twenty years. I still have 10,000 followers on my FaceBook page but get shut down if I mention anything about vaccines, COVID or related topics. This just another indication of how the current medical mafia is protecting their turf. Another example of how our 1st Amendment rights have being eroded away and violated by big corporate monopoly's.

Many of the studies that I have in my research data have been removed from the internet and journaled studies have been hidden. It is difficult to find any information that goes against the vaccine narrative. The good news is my 6-part DVD series, VACCINES: Risks, Responsibility and Rights, has all the references from journals, studies, research stats and even the CDC charts documenting my vaccine statements and research.

This series covers from the polio era to the cervical cancer vaccine era. It does not cover the COVID pandemic or thee covid injections. We are still learning about the COVID gene therapies and they are even more diabolical than the previous vaccines. They are not immunizations; they are a genetic therapy designed to track those who take it and much more.

I recently published a PDF file called, <u>COVID Pandemic Exposed</u>. This report is available by download from my website for a small fee. As scientists, doctors and researchers began to examine people who suffered injury or died post-vaccine, we began to see a glimpse of the physical and emotional consequences. Some it was the initial jab and for others it was the boosters. Not only did they discover that the jab did not protect but thousands were reinfected with the COVID illness.

This report will expose what scientists are finding in the COVID-19 injection vials (not vaccines), created in the lab that are completely artificial and have artificial intelligence. Many scientists and physicians were curious as to why the injections had to be frozen at 90 degrees, sub-zero temperatures until use. The vials from the different manufactures have been carefully thawed and examined to discover what is in these jabs. When vials reach body temperature, a group of doctors photographed and documented creepy parasitic-like critters that resemble known parasites or "new" lab-created monsters. These foreign critters grow and develop long tentacles and even a "foot" to help them manipulate around in the body! These critters may be responsible for the huge clotting problem killing young athletes and causing heart attacks referred to as Myocarditis and Pericarditis after receiving the mRNA COVID – 19 vaccines. I call this jab a "Clot Shot" because they are causing huge clot issues also verified by funeral directors!

My report is currently 60 pages of documentation about masks, outlawed medications, school and church shut-downs, and hospital procedures that are killing people and the fallout of death and injury post COVID – 19 shots, available on my website, http://www.ChildhoodShots.com

Chapter 11

The True Purpose of Well-Baby Visits

A famous pediatrician, Dr. Robert Mendelsohn, wrote a profound book, "How to Raise a Healthy Child in Spite of your Doctor." Dr. Mendelsohn focuses on supporting new parents by educating them on the "normal childhood illnesses" and guides them on how to treat their children at home safely. Obviously, from the title of his book, he does not encourage the frequent use of pediatricians, and he writes that "the purpose of the pediatrician is to indoctrinate your child into a life-long dependency on drugs…the well-baby visit is worthless."[22]

Prior to the 1970s, Americans had a general practitioner who was either a MD (medical doctor) or a DO (doctor of osteopathy). One only saw the doctor if ill and a few vaccines were administered between the ages of four and five years old. This differs greatly with what happens today when one thinks of the average American pediatrician. Statistically, American children were healthier back in the 1970s than they are now. There were no pediatric cancer wards in every hospital, no asthma centers in every city; children did not suffer with chronic ear infections requiring ear tube surgery. Children did not have Type 2 diabetes, learning problems, ADD, ADHD, obesity, and they did not go to their pediatrician when healthy.

---

[22] Mendelsohn, Robert S. "How to Raise a Healthy Child in Spite of your Doctor: One of America's Leading Pediatricians Puts Parents Back in Control of Their Children's Health." *Ballantine Books.* May 12, 1987.

The American Academy of Pediatrics recommends babies receive checkups at birth, 3 to 5 days after birth and then at 1,2,4,6,9,12,15,18 and 24 months. The well baby visit is entirely about ensuring the child is up to date on vaccines. To confirm this, a simple Google search of "well-baby visit" shows it exclusively focuses on the ever-growing vaccine schedule.

In my opinion, pediatrician visits are for sick children; healthy children do not need medical care. Parents know when their children are sick and when they are not. They do not need for a doctor that barely knows their child to tell them so. Furthermore, the pediatrician's office is full of vaccinated children who may be contagious; putting your child at an increased risk. It has been proven that live virus vaccines "shed" for up to three months after they are administered, so recently vaccinated people can *spread* the illness. This is true for the FluMist Quadrivalent Influenza vaccine, the MMR vaccine (measles, mumps and rubella), the Varicella vaccine (chickenpox), the RotaTeq vaccine (rotavirus), and Zostavax (shingles). This shedding effect is especially prevalent in the vaccine recommended for family members of newborn babies: the TDaP vaccine (diphtheria, whooping cough and tetanus). [23]

A 2000 study in the Journal of Emerging Infections Diseases concluded that "vaccinated adolescents and adults may serve as reservoirs for silent infections and become potential transmitters to unprotected infants. The whole-cell vaccine for Pertussis is protective only against clinical disease, not against infection. Even young, recently vaccinated children (and adults) may serve as reservoirs and potential transmitters of

---

[23] Warfel, Jason M., Zimmerman, Lindsay L. and Merkel, Tod J. "Acellular Pertussis Vaccines Protect Against Disease But Fail to Prevent Infection and Transmission in a Nonhuman Primate Model." *Proceedings of the National Academy of Sciences USA.* January 14, 2014.

infection."[24] Mainstream media would have people believe that it is the unvaccinated children who are spreading diseases such as measles and whooping cough, but this simply isn't true. These illnesses are occurring in children who have been fully vaccinated!

In many instances, parents feel more at ease having a pediatrician available in the chance that one is needed. I encourage parents to find one that respects their medical decisions for their child and does not make the parent feel guilty or negligent about their choices. If a pediatrician refuses to care for a child because of the parents' choice to not vaccinate, I recommend the parents find a doctor who will respect their healthcare choices. There are pediatricians who will not force the vaccine issue. Medical freedom groups, vaccine rights groups, mommy groups, midwives and chiropractors can be a great referral source for these physicians. I advise parents to be prepared when going into a pediatrician's office. When I was part of a nationally syndicated vaccine seminar, that health departments from across the county were required to participate in, I was surprised to discover the tactics used by medical practices in vaccination indoctrination. They use slick psychological methods to persuade parents who are unsure to agree to vaccinating. Do your research, make your decision and be prepared.

The pediatricians have overseen the health of American children for the last 50 years. During this time, the health of children has declined. This should be a huge red flag for anyone promoting this type of healthcare. When looking at the statistics below, it is important to mention that perhaps some

---

[4] Miller, Neil Z., and Goldman, Gary S. "Infant Mortality Rates Regressed Against Number of Vaccine Doses Routinely Given: Is there a Biochemical or Synergistic Toxicity?" *Sage Journals*. May 4, 2011.

of these conditions were overlooked in previous years, but even that would not compensate for the vast difference.

1960 – 3% of children chronic illness, 97% of children healthy
1970 – 6% of children chronic illness, 94% of children healthy
1994 – 12% of children chronic illness, 88% of children healthy
2006 – 26% of children chronic illness, 74% of children healthy
2011 – 54% of children chronically ill with asthma, diabetes, learning problems, severe food allergies, autism, ADHD, ADD, depression, autoimmune illnesses, seizure disorders, cancers, blindness and hearing loss and obesity, with most requiring daily medication.

The devastating fact is that less than half of the pediatric population is healthy. The National Survey of Children's Health from May-June 2011 estimated that 32 million children had at least *1 of 20 chronic health conditions* assessed, increasing to 54.1% when overweight, obese, or being at risk for developmental delays were included. Furthermore:
In 2012 – 1 in 88 diagnosed with autism spectrum disorder
By 2017 – 1 in 36 diagnosed with autism spectrum disorder

According to a report performed in 2017, the United States has the worst overall child mortality rate compared with those of 19 other wealthy nations. Dr. Ashish Thakrar, the lead author of the study and an internal medicine resident at Johns Hopkins Hospital states, "This study should alarm everyone. The US is the most dangerous of wealthy, democratic countries in the world for children," He continues, "We were surprised by how far the US has fallen behind other wealthy countries. Across all ages and in both sexes, children have been dying more often in the US than in similar countries since the 1980s."[25]

A 2011 study done by Neil Z. Miller and Gary S. Goldman in the Human and Experimental Toxicology: SAGE Journal, confirms that "full-term infants in the US were anywhere from 50 percent to 200 percent more likely to die within the first year of life than infants in Austria, Denmark, Finland, Norway, Sweden, and Switzerland, depending on the state."[26] In this country vaccinations are the backbone of the childhood health program. We administer two times more vaccines than most other countries and yet our children become unhealthier as each year passes and we have higher death rates for the first year of life. These statistics confirm a failed childhood healthcare system. A healthcare system that is built on the foundation of vaccinations. It is evident that this foundation destroys health for a large segment of the population.

"The greatest threat to childhood diseases lies in the dangerous and ineffectual efforts made to prevent them through mass immunization...There is no convincing scientific evidence that mass inoculations can be credited with eliminating any childhood disease."
-Dr. Robert Mendelsohn

---

[25] Howard, Jacqueline. "Among 20 wealthy nations, US child mortality ranks worst, study finds". CNN health. January 8,2018. https://www.cnn.com/2018/01/08/health/child-mortality-rates-by-country-study-intl/index.html.

[26] Miller, Neil Z., and Goldman, Gary S. "Infant Mortality Rates Regressed Against Number of Vaccine Doses Routinely Given: Is there a Biochemical or Synergistic Toxicity?" *Sage Journals.* May 4, 2011.

"The doctor of the future will give no medicine but will interest his patients in the care of the human frame, in diet and in the cause and prevention of disease." -Thomas Edison

Chapter 12

The Healing Journey

If you or your child suffer with vaccine injuries, I would like you to know that there is hope. There have been many advancements in the natural healthcare field, and in many cases, progress can be made. For some, this progress means better behavior, less symptoms, less food sensitivities, better quality of life, and in some miraculous instances, complete recovery of vaccine injury. There are many considerations that factor into the recovery process including: the severity of injury, how much time has passed since the injury occurred, lifestyle, age, past medical treatments, medications, and genetics. I encourage parents not to wait. The sooner intervention can take place the better.

I have been blessed to learn from and work with many advanced physicians who have dedicated their lives to helping people of all ages with vaccine injuries. My daughter, Renee Hunter D.C. was trained as a Defeat Autism Now (DAN) physician in 2007. This training program was started by Bernard Rimland who had a son with autism. He was a psychologist, writer, lecturer, founder and director of two advocacy groups: The Autism Society of America (ASA) and the Autism Research Institute (ARI). People who closely worked with him say he was responsible for helping over 1500 children recover from regressive autism. Dr. Rimland hypothesized that children with autism had weakened immune systems and fragile digestive systems. He believed that environmental pollutants, antibiotics and toxic vaccine metals like thimerosal (mercury) were responsible for destroying beneficial bacteria. Thousands of functional doctors have validated his conclusion through lab testing. As expected, traditional doctors have not only tried to discredit him, but firmly state that autism cannot be reversed. They are just plain wrong. I encourage you to YouTube Dominic's Autism Recovery Journey and Oscar Recovering through the Son-Rise Program. These are just a few of thousands who have seen great results using various treatment protocols. I am careful to never use the word "cure", but I have seen individuals with severe autism (limited to no communication skills, poor to no eye contact, poor posture, shy and anti-social behavior, refusal to eat vegetables, stimming and compulsive behavior, dark circles around eyes, bloated abdomen, skin rashes, and sensory processing issues) make great progress and become highly functional. Unfortunately, the DAN doctors training program was infiltrated by Johnson & Johnson and eventually shut down. Another example of big pharma destroying any opportunity to help recover children. Now, parents must seek out a new type of doctor called "functional" medical doctors who specialize in autism spectrum disorders. This field in medicine is made of physicians who are aware of the causes and have branched out away from traditional allopathic medicine, and have specialized training in natural modalities. They can offer hope to families.

Between the years of 2009-2012, my daughter Renee, Karen Hubert, CNHP (Certified Natural Health Professional), NC (Nutritional Consultant), and I, held five training conferences for physicians called, "Hope for Autism". The conferences were focused on not only understanding what occurred during vaccine injury, but also treatment protocols to reverse the damage. At least 12 different doctors who all specialized in various aspects of holistic healing were in attendance and presented. In attendance, were also functional medical doctors, researchers, authors, pediatric chiropractors, naturopathic physicians, pediatric gastroenterologists, heavy metal experts, MD brain experts, early child development experts, immunologists, neurologists, and food sensitivity allergy experts. These conferences filled me with hope for those who had been injured by vaccines.

There was a family I knew that had three vaccine injured children. Their oldest son, who had the most severe symptoms, started his recovery journey three years before we began holding our conferences. His mother would not only show pictures of her children, but described them as unwell with distended bellies, highly allergic to foods, antisocial behavior, stunted communication and language skills, and chronically sick. With treatments, her eldest son continued to get better with each passing year. On the last day of our conference, he was our final speaker. With great confidence and clarity, he shared, in detail, how it felt to be stuck in autism prior to his recovery. Charmingly, he connected with the audience and encouraged our newly trained doctors to get out there and reach other injured children. There wasn't a dry eye in the room, and we all knew there was hope in vaccine injury recovery.

Many physicians are learning about natural protocols to reverse not only vaccine injury, but many chronic illnesses and health challenges. This specialized field is ever-expanding and as I stated before, they are called Functional Medical doctors. They are trying to help the demands of our sick nation. I am not a licensed healthcare professional or a doctor, but I have learned about advanced medical protocols and natural treatments to help the healing process. I have been exposed to the newest testing and various protocols offered. Although each case is different, there are a few key points that apply to all. First, I firmly believe in testing… not guessing. There are so many valuable specialized tests available. There are tests that can evaluate the GI tract and assess for microbial imbalances, tests that can identify nutritional deficiencies, food allergies and sensitivities, environmental allergens, inflammation in the body, antibody issues, heavy metal toxicity, hidden infections, hormonal imbalances and much more. A trained physician can help determine which tests will be most beneficial. Taking supplements and following protocols without first assessing the body is dangerous and frequently leads to wasted time and money. It is important to state that each person is uniquely different. One man's medicine is another man's poison.

It is not only good to have a baseline of how the body is at the beginning of treatment, but follow-up testing is also advised to assess progress and determine if treatments need to be altered. Due to restrictions from the insurance companies, I have found that many of these alternative physicians do not participate with insurance and work on a cash basis. In rare instances, insurance may cover lab testing and some physicians may bill insurance. For those unsure of where to start or in need of guidance when choosing a doctor, I am available for consultations. Although I do not make medical recommendations, I can help to provide assistance in choosing the right physician and information for various lab testing, protocols and natural substances (visit my website for scheduling).

The second thing I highly recommend to everyone is to keep detailed journal or log of all symptoms, treatments and progress. This is easy as it costs no money and takes just a little bit of time. Frequently throughout a healing journey, it is easy to forget beginning symptoms and the severity of those symptoms. Keeping a detailed log helps to not only provide important information regarding progress, but lets you know when you are on the right track. Even small steps in the right direction can make a huge impact! Healing takes time and unfortunately, there are no quick, easy fixes.

Although many parents have had great success with natural self-guided treatment protocols, I encourage people to work with a trained physician. In the long run this can save suffering and money. Many different types of doctors offer specialized testing and healing protocols. It could be a naturopathic physician, a chiropractor, a nurse practitioner, a functional medicine doctor, or a holistic physician that guides the healing journey. Whatever the health issues are, there is always progress to be made. For some, this progress will be huge and offer life changing results. There is nothing more beautiful than seeing health recovery in another.

"Education is the most powerful weapon which you can use to change the world." -Nelson Mandela

Chapter 13

The Vaccine Education Revolution

I coined the term, "The Vaccine Education Revolution," over twenty-five years ago when I first began lecturing on this topic. Now more than ever, parents, doctors, scientists, and activists are speaking out about the dark side of vaccinations. These individuals do not choose to fight this politically-incorrect battle for no good reason. In most cases, they have witnessed the damaging effects of vaccines and have become outraged with the industries blatant disregard and massive cover-up of those who have been injured.

Most parents are stunned to find thousands of others with very similar stories surrounding vaccine injury. When someone suffers vaccine injury themselves or has a child that was injured, it can be a very confusing and overwhelming time. The sad part is that parents are often doing what they think it right for their child. They are told that good parents take their children in for well-baby visits and that their health and life depends on being up to date on vaccinations. The chance of adverse health reactions or injury is not considered because it is not openly disclosed. I often wonder, if doctors openly discussed the potential side effects with parents, how many would choose to forgo the vaccine? How many parents would vaccinate with the chickenpox vaccine (Varivax) if they knew potential side effects were encephalitis, meningitis, Bell's palsy or anaphylaxis? I have a feeling that most parents would take their chance with chicken pox, a normal childhood disease in which "pox parties" were once quite common.

Individuals who were once firm believers in vaccinations and have seen the unshared side of this practice, are the ones who are fueling the movement of non-vaccinators (or as many people call them antivaxxers). Unfortunately, these people are often publicly ridiculed, attacked by the vaccine industry, have their professional careers destroyed, are called irresponsible, evil, and are even blamed for outbreaks. On quite a few occasions, I have been referred to as an "anti-vaccine liar" even though the information I present is based on hard peer-reviewed science. In my lectures, I reference over 15 medical journals and present graphs and charts compiled by the CDC. These are the consequences for going against the grain and standing up to a multi-billion-dollar industry.

In an indoctrinated society, the act of researching and questioning comes to a halt. I am elated that so many are breaking free of this indoctrination and are leading this vaccine education revolution. It is time that all aspects of vaccinations, including adverse reactions and vaccine ineffectiveness are disclosed, openly discussed and researched. It also needs to be public knowledge that the US has a court system dedicated to vaccine injury. Established in 1986, the US Court of Federal Claims is a no-fault system protecting Big Pharma from all financial liability. The settlement money comes from a $0.75 tax on every vaccine given. The court decides who deserves compensation for vaccine injury and death with a financial cap for death of a person at $250,000. Below are some of the stats from the US Court of Federal Claims from 2014-2015.[27]

---

[27] Gregory, Lauren Martin. "US Vax Court Sees 400% Increase in Vaccine Injury Payouts, Flu Shot Wins Top Honor for Biggest Payout". The Mom Street Journal. November 26,2016. https://www.themomstreetjournal.com/increase-in-vaccine-injury-payouts/.

Vaccine court settlement payouts increased in total from $22.8 million in 2014 to $114 million in 2015 — a $400% increase.

Some specific examples:
The most expensive payout in 2015 was for influenza vaccine injuries. In 2014 they paid out $4.9 million and in 2015 they paid out $61 million — this is over a 1000% increase.

Varicella (chickenpox) has the third largest increase in payouts from $0 in 2014 to $5.8 million in 2015.

Payouts for death and injuries from the Hepatitis B vaccine was the fourth largest increase in court settlements with payouts from $1.9 million in 2014 to $8 million in 2015 — a 321% increase.

Injury payout from the TDaP/DTP/DPT and D/T were the fifth largest increase from $5.5 million in 2014 to $9.8 million in 2015 — a 75% increase.

The Special Masters of the US Court of Federal Claims are given full authority as judge and jury to decide compensation for those who feel they have been injured by vaccines. Every January, this non-traditional court releases an annual report, providing the public with a peek into its inner workings. This report is consistently ignored by health officials, politicians, mainstream media and the CDC. In fact, I would be willing to wager that over 90% of Americans do not know this court exists. Even Nancy Grace, a top TV attorney was shocked to learn of this secret no-fault court system when she was interviewing the mother of a teen boy who died after the flu vaccine. These settlement statistics should outrage and shock everyone. These statistics are from adults and children injured or killed by vaccines. The same vaccines that are promoted as safe and effective, and in many states, are being forced upon people; whether they want them or not.

It is our duty as humans to warn others of the potential harm associated with vaccines. It is our duty to break free from the indoctrination and be willing to go against the grain. It is our duty to protect our children. There are many ways one can get involved with Vaccine Education Revolution such as: Hosting a "Watch party" in your home and share my DVD series, especially Part 3 where I expose toxic ingredients. Join local groups dedicated to vaccine education and natural healthcare, hosting lectures in your community, or participating in local events aimed at vaccine choice. I highly recommend everyone become familiar with their states vaccine exemptions and get involved with state groups focused on protecting medical freedom. Not only do these groups need financial support, but also participation from people who understand the value to having medical freedom of choice.

"There is no such thing as freedom of choice unless there is freedom to refuse." -David Hume

You either promote health, or by default, you produce disease.

Author Unknown

Chapter 14

Not Vaccinating is Not Enough

In today's extremely toxic world, not vaccinating is not enough. Toxins are prevalent in our air, food, water, cleaning supplies, furniture, and personal care products. The human body has detox pathways in place to handle toxins, but when exposure gets too high or the pathways aren't working well, the body can become overloaded. There are hundreds of adverse health effects that may arise from exposures to toxins. These potential effects include cancer, high blood pressure, asthma, deficits in attention, memory, learning, IQ, Parkinson's-like diseases, infertility, shortened lactation, endometriosis, genital malformation, peripheral nerve damage, and dysfunctional immune systems. Developing or immature tissues are far more susceptible to toxic exposures than adult tissues. This means developing fetuses and children are far more sensitive to toxic chemical exposure. There are also some toxins that are harder for the body to eliminate. For anyone wanting to promote health, eliminating exposure to toxins is an absolute necessity.

The first place to start is in the home. Ensuring that foods eaten are organic and whole with a focus on minimizing any processed or unhealthy foods. Traditional food is laden with pesticides, insecticides, herbicides, fungicides, glyphosate

"Roundup", artificial coloring, and genetically modified organisms. Every bite of food either promotes disease or health, so choose wisely. Another major area of concern is toxic water. Industrial dumping, pesticide runoff, leaky storage tanks, and governmental mandates have created big water problems. Common water contaminates include: Fluoride, chlorine, lead, arsenic and dioxins. A healthy water source such as Berkey water filtration is ideal in removing toxins and ensuring safe drinking water.

Personal care products are also a key area for concern. A study conducted in 2014, found that the average person is exposed to more than a hundred chemicals from cosmetics, soaps and other personal care products before leaving the house in the morning.[28] There are currently 11,700 chemicals used in personal care products that are registered with the Environmental Protection Agency. These chemicals can enter the body by either penetrating the skin or being inhaled throughout the day. Simply choosing non-toxic organic personal care products can help reduce this toxic load tremendously. There are also some great do-it-yourself personal care products online.

Another large source for toxic chemical exposure is home cleaning products. There are 84,000 industrial chemicals used in household items. Of these, only 200 have been tested by the FDA, only 5 are regulated by the FDA and the last time

---

[28] Roeder, Amy. "Harmful, untested chemicals rife in personal care products". Harvard T.H. Chan School of Public Health. 2014.
https://www.hsph.harvard.edu/news/features/harmful-chemicals-in-personal-care-products/.

federal chemical safety law was updated was in 1976. [29] Toxicity ranges from corrosive chemicals used in oven cleaners to major hormone disrupters and cancer causers in dryer sheets and laundry detergents. When in doubt, go with non-toxic organic products for in-home use. There are also many resources online for making your own cleaners. I encourage people to use up what you have and systematically, replace with clean, natural products! You may spend a little more but the investment will help save you pain and suffering in your future.

Eating organic foods will help support a natural, strong immune system in addition, reduce the toxic load you carry. If you have young children, please purchase natural foods for them while they are developing their brain and organs. Even if you cannot afford to feed everyone organic foods, at least provide them for your young children. School lunchroom food is terrible! Most packaged foods in schools are microwaved and highly processed with very little nutritional value! Do your best to send kids off to school with a lunch packed from home supplying them the nutrition their brains and bodies need for learning and growing. I hope to see this process-food trend in schools changed as parents get involved and demand higher quality foods for the developing brains.

In addition to making sure the home is a safe and healthy environment, I am also a huge proponent of chiropractic care for the whole family. I have been under chiropractic care for over 40 years and found it to be an integral part of raising a healthy family, naturally. My ex-husband is a chiropractor and I have two daughters who are also doctors of chiropractic. I have witnessed the ability that chiropractic care has in bringing

---

[29] Urbina, Ian. "Think Those Chemicals Have Been Tested?". The New York times. April 13, 2012. https://www.nytimes.com/2013/04/14/sunday-review/think-those-chemicals-have-been-tested.html.

harmony and healing to the body. It focuses on restoring proper function and communication throughout the body and is a must have tool needed for raising healthy children. I view Chiropractors as the "mechanics" for the body. They carefully remove interferences in the nervous system that reduce function. By removing these interferences, the body can function at its optimum level. Chiropractic care is also important for children. Many times, throughout birth, especially with children born via C-Section, there can be trauma to the cervical neck. This trauma, if left untreated, can lead to many issues including stomach issues, sleeping problems, ear infections and much more. Chiropractic has been proven safe for babies and children. I recommend researching chiropractic health benefits and finding a good family chiropractor who will support a natural health approach.

Choosing natural options from conception to birth will provide an advantage for children, but proactive approaches are needed to facilitate and maintain health throughout life. One must be equipped with practical tools needed as normal childhood health conditions arise. Common childhood problems may include ear infections, sore throats, croupy coughs, headaches, skin rashes, body pains, swollen glands, nausea, fevers and runny noses. It is always better to start learning various methods to dealing with these illnesses before you are presented with them. Being properly equipped also means knowing what to do if in a crisis; getting a good foundation under your belt for those trying times when you may need a medical doctor. There are so many wonderful resources available today for parents. Websites dedicated to natural plant-based products designed to help the body during times of illness and books devoted to education and natural remedies. Now more than ever there is easy access to chiropractors, naturopathic physicians, homeopathic physicians, holistic nurse practitioners, nutritionists and even functional medical doctors who are practicing holistic medicine. There are also natural support groups which can often be a source of encouragement, information and wisdom.

My hope is that you will respect the innate wisdom that governs us all; allowing it to work without interference as much as possible. With knowledge and support, comes the ability to know when the body needs to be left alone to work and learn how to defend itself, and when medical intervention is needed.

I pray this information has been helpful to you and your family. I hope you have learned a lot and are better prepared to live well and raise naturally healthy children. I believe God has given us all the tools needed to live a happy healthy life, we just need to know how to use them.

May you and your family be blessed!

Future book subjects in this series:

Birthing Options and Outcomes
Raising Healthy Families in a Toxic World
Creating Fabulous Health in Your Senior Years
The Vaccine Education Revolution

Made in the USA
Middletown, DE
Updated 2022 October 24

Made in the USA
Monee, IL
29 July 2023

40083643R00059